EVALUATING THE MEDICAL CARE SYSTEM

Lu Ann Aday

Charles E. Begley

David R. Lairson

Carl H. Slater

EVALUATING THE MEDICAL CARE SYSTEM

Effectiveness, Efficiency, and Equity

Health Administration Press
Ann Arbor, Michigan   1993

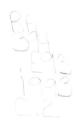

97 96 95 94 93   5 4 3 2 1

Library of Congress Cataloging-in-Publication Data

Evaluating the medical care system : effectiveness, efficiency, and equity / Lu Ann Aday . . . [et al.].
    p.   cm.
  Includes bibliographical references and index.
  ISBN 0910701989 (softbound : alk. paper)
  1. Medical care—Evaluation.   2. Medical care—Research.   3. Medical policy—Evaluation.   I. Aday, Lu Ann.
  [DNLM: 1. Delivery of Health Care—United States.   2. Health Services Research—United States.   3. Health Policy—United States.   W 84 AA1 E85 1993]
RA394.E93   1993   362.1'068'5—dc20
DNLM/DLC for Library of Congress   93-20495 CIP

The paper used in this publication meets the minimum requirements of American National Standard for Information Sciences—Permanence of Paper for Printed Library Materials, ANSI Z39.48-1984. ∞™

Health Administration Press
A division of the Foundation of the
  American College of Healthcare
  Executives
1021 East Huron Street
Ann Arbor, Michigan 48104-9990
(313) 764-1380

The Association for Health
  Services Research
1350 Connecticut Avenue, NW
Suite 1100
Washington, DC 20036
(202) 223-2477

Contents

List of Figures and Tables

Figures

Tables

Foreword

In many respects, those who seek to understand the U.S. health care system and U.S. health care policy are like the blind persons who try to describe the proverbial elephant based on the part that they alone "observe." In a country as diverse as the United States, both health services delivery and health care policymaking are complex processes that cannot be fully understood from any single perspective. Revealing and connecting the components of the health care system in the context of the whole is one of the valuable roles of health services research.

With the publication of *Evaluating the Medical Care System: Effectiveness, Efficiency, and Equity*, we now have three volumes that shed light on the contributions of health services research to public policy. Eli Ginzberg's edited volume, *Health Services Research: Key to Health Policy* (1991), summarizes the many contributions of health services research over the past two decades. The Baxter Health Policy Review book, *Improving Health Policy and Management: Nine Critical Research Issues for the 1990s* (1992), provides cogent summaries and discussions of recent, ongoing, and evolving research targeted to specific current policy issues, ranging from the design of a core health benefit package to issues surrounding the prolongation of life. And this book, by Lu Ann Aday, Charles E. Begley, David R. Lairson, and Carl H. Slater, provides an extremely useful bridge between the Ginzberg and Baxter volumes by offering a conceptual framework for thinking about the issues and providing some detail on the tools (methods and data bases) that health services and health policy researchers use in carrying out their work.

A major strength of this book is that the authors have evolved a holistic and integrative vision of the "health care elephant" as viewed through the lenses of the effectiveness, efficiency, and equity concepts. Within each of these domains the major issues, concepts, methods, and evidence are presented from multiple perspectives. For example, effectiveness issues are considered from both an overall population-based focus and an individual clinical perspective. Issues of efficiency are considered from both an allocative social welfare perspective and a production theory of the firm perspective. Equity of access issues are addressed from approaches based on entitlement and needs, and from egalitarian, contractarian, and utilitarian approaches. In each case and from each perspective, relevant data are marshalled to enable readers to understand the current state of knowledge regarding the issue at hand. In addition, the data and evidence illuminate such current health policy issues as the development, dissemination, and implementation of practice guidelines, physician payment reform (e.g., RBRVS), and proposals for health care reform.

The authors are to be particularly commended for their discussion of the types of health services research that can best influence different stages of the policy process. The strengths and limitations of the rational-comprehensive, satisficing, mixed-scanning, and political models of policymaking are also duly noted. The utility of the overall framework of effectiveness, efficiency, and equity is illustrated in reviewing major approaches to health care reform, including the Canadian-style single payer model, consumer choice plans, and the Pepper Commission's mixed regulatory-competitive approach.

In the final analysis, this is an exemplar of truly integrative work. Superbly organized and clearly written, it is of equal value to researchers, policymakers, and those involved in the direct provision and management of health services delivery. This book makes a significant contribution toward the development of a common language and knowledge base for anyone interested in improving the performance of the U.S. medical care system.

Stephen M. Shortell
A. C. Buehler Distinguished Professor
   of Health Services Management and
Professor of Organization Behavior
J. L. Kellogg Graduate School of Management
Center for Health Services and Policy Research
Northwestern University
Evanston, Illinois

Preface

This book defines and integrates the fundamental concepts and methods of health services research as a field of study, and illustrates their application to policy analysis. A model of health policy analysis is linked to a framework for classifying topics and issues in health services research. The book provides a historical perspective and applies the concepts and methods of epidemiology, economics, sociology, and related disciplines to illustrate the measurement and relevance of effectiveness, efficiency, and equity as criteria for evaluating health care system performance. Specific examples of the application of health services research in addressing contemporary health policy problems at the national, state, and local levels are presented.

The primary audiences for the book are practicing professionals and graduate students in public health, health administration, and the health care professions, and federal, state, and local policymakers and program planners charged with the design and conduct of policy-relevant health services research. Professionals and students in medical sociology, the behavioral sciences, and public administration interested in conducting applied or policy-oriented health and health care research will also find the book of considerable interest. The authors developed and applied the perspective presented in the book in a course they have offered to master's and doctoral students in public health since 1986.

Chapter 1 presents a framework for classifying the major topics and issues addressed by health services research as a field of study. This framework is then utilized to provide an integrative overview of the contributions of health services research to describing and evaluating the performance of the medical care system with respect to the objectives of effectiveness, efficiency, and equity. This chapter defines the relationship between health services research and the major objectives and methods of policy analysis. The historical role of health services research in the formulation of health policy is highlighted.

Chapter 2 deals with the effectiveness of medical care in terms of the contribution medical care makes to health and whether that contribution can be enhanced. A conceptual framework based on Donabedian's classical triad of structure, process, and outcome, and the associated methods for assessing the effectiveness of medical care at both the population and clinical levels, are presented. Chapter 3 reviews the evidence derived from studies using these methods and explores the role of effectiveness research in developing clinical practice guidelines.

Chapter 4 examines the concepts of production and allocative efficiency and the empirical methods for assessing each. Chapter 5 discusses the major findings regarding the performance of the U.S. medical care system with respect to these objectives, and describes the past and future role of efficiency analysis in physician payment reform.

Chapter 6 introduces the concept of equity of access to medical care in the context of the theoretical and ethical considerations underlying a right to medical care. An empirical approach for evaluating the extent to which alternative norms of fairness have been achieved is introduced. Chapter 7 summarizes empirical data documenting the current performance of the medical care delivery system with respect to equity. A final section of the chapter introduces the issue of universal health insurance and the contributions of health services research to assessing the potential of such a mechanism for improving access.

Chapter 8 analyzes the interrelationships between and among the objectives of effectiveness, efficiency, and equity, and the role of health services research in conceptualizing and measuring the trade-offs among them in formulating health policy. Chapter 9 discusses these trade-offs in the context of evaluating specific universal health insurance alternatives.

The unique contributions this book makes are: (1) it presents and applies an organizing framework for defining health services research as a field of study, in the context of the major system performance dimensions of effectiveness, efficiency, and equity; (2) it reviews and integrates the conceptual, methodological, and empirical contributions of health services research to addressing these issues; (3) it illustrates how the perspectives and methods of effectiveness, efficiency, and equity research can be used to anticipate and pose relevant questions to inform both current and future health care policy debates; and (4) it provides a primer and point of reference at a time when both the support for and demands upon health services research and policy analysis are increasing.

Lu Ann Aday
Charles E. Begley
David R. Lairson
Carl H. Slater

Acknowledgments

The authors gratefully acknowledge colleagues, Stephen H. Linder and David Colby, as well as the anonymous Health Administration Press reviewers, who provided thoughtful and constructive comments on earlier drafts of the manuscript.

Special thanks go to Adel Youssef and Chih-Wen Chung, who located and copied many of the sources cited in the book, and to Regina Fisher, Lawana Norris, and Doris Ross, who assisted with typing the manuscript.

We are grateful for the flexible environment at the University of Texas School of Public Health, which supported the rewarding task of writing the book as a routine component of faculty roles and responsibilities.

We owe a special debt to the students in our course on Health Services Delivery and Performance throughout the years, as well as to students in Carl Slater's Medical Outcomes Assessment class, who stimulated and challenged us to sharpen our mastery of the ideas put forth in the book.

Each of us feels that our understanding of the concepts of effectiveness, efficiency, and equity has been broadened and deepened in the process of writing the book. Our hope is that those who read it will be similarly rewarded.

Chapter 1

Introduction to Health Services Research and Policy Analysis

Definitions

Health services research *produces* knowledge about the performance of the medical care system, and policy analysis *applies* this knowledge in defining problems and evaluating policy alternatives. This book delineates and defines the working partnership between health services research and policy analysis in assessing the performance of the U.S. medical care system with respect to the objectives of effectiveness, efficiency, and equity, where

1. *effectiveness* concerns the benefits of medical care measured by improvements in health;
2. *efficiency* relates these health improvements to the resources required to produce them; and
3. *equity* assesses whether the benefits and burdens of medical care are fairly distributed.

The *effectiveness* of medical care concerns the benefits of medical care as measured by *improvements in people's health*. Improvements in health not only include the sum of the individual benefits, that is, reduced mortality rates, increased life expectancies, and the decreased prevalence of disease, but also refer to a distribution of disease and health such that overall economic productivity and well-being are maximized.

A second major objective of the health care delivery system is the drive for *efficiency*. Where medical care is viewed as an output, we are concerned about *production efficiency* (producing services at least cost), and where medical care is viewed as an input in the production of health improvements, we are concerned with *allocative efficiency* (maximizing health given constrained resources).[1] Allocative efficiency depends on the relative cost and effectiveness of medical care in improving health. Ultimately, maximization of health requires both production and allocative efficiency.

Equity is concerned with the fair distribution of the benefits and burdens (including the costs) of medical care among groups or individuals. What is fair will differ, depending on the values that are used in making these judgments. For some, the personal freedom to choose from a number of different options and to decide the kind of care they want without being dictated to by anyone else is of utmost importance. Others would define fairness norms more in terms of the costs and outcomes for different people or society as a whole: Is everyone being treated equally? Are those who need it most being helped? Is the well-being of society as a whole enhanced? Are the benefits on average for each person maximized? Allocative efficiency most closely operationalizes these last two norms of fairness, particularly in the context of constrained resources. Which norm ultimately prevails in formulating health policy is largely a function of its dominance in the political arena.

There are two ways of relating the effectiveness, efficiency, and equity objectives. One is to attempt to determine which is a better criterion in evaluating the performance of the health care system. This is a normative question that is subject to differing views of the nature of medical care and the role of the health care system. Its answer is best left to the political process. The second way is in terms of observable relations. This question can be addressed by health services research that identifies how these objectives complement or conflict with each other. Our primary focus is on the second question in the context of identifying the empirical trade-offs among the effectiveness, efficiency, and equity objectives.

The three objectives are often complementary. Improving medical care effectiveness while holding resources constant increases efficiency. Increases in efficiency create opportunities for improved effectiveness and equity. However, the objectives may also be in conflict. Maximizing effectiveness by allocating additional resources to improve health may conflict with efficiency if the cost of the resources is very high relative to their effectiveness. Maximizing effectiveness and efficiency by distributing resources to persons who would gain most may be inequitable if the policy leads to a very uneven distribution.

Identifying appropriate trade-offs among the three objectives is an important product of health services research. Assuming that all three are important objectives, a key question for decision makers in comparing policy alternatives is the degree to which one objective must be sacrificed to achieve the others.

The chapters that follow review the conceptual, methodological, and empirical foundations for the effectiveness, efficiency, and equity objectives, show how they are applied in policy analysis, and examine the health services research questions posed in analyzing the trade-offs between these objectives in formulating health policy.

In this chapter, the fields of health services research and policy analysis are compared and contrasted with other types of inquiry. A framework for classifying topics and issues in health services research is presented and used to provide a descriptive overview of the U.S. medical care system. Historical contributions of health services research to the development of health policy are highlighted, and selected applications in terms of current U.S. policy debates are introduced.

Definition of health services research

A 1979 Institute of Medicine panel charged with defining and evaluating the field of health services research offered the following definition of the enterprise: "Health services research is inquiry to produce knowledge about the structure, processes or effects of personal health services" (Institute of Medicine 1979, 14). A study could be classified as health services research if it dealt primarily with "personal health services" and drew upon a conceptual framework other than that of applied biomedical science (that primarily focuses on the fundamental life processes of the human organism). Personal health services are transactions between providers and clients for the purpose of promoting the health of the clients. These transactions largely fall within the domain of the *medical care* system, in contrast to *public health* which focuses on interventions to promote the health and well-being of the community or population as a whole, rather than particular individuals within it.

Health services research is inherently *inter*disciplinary in focus, in that it draws upon and applies theories and methods from an array of disciplines, including sociology, political science, epidemiology, demography, economics, and law, among others (Choi and Greenberg 1982). Basic disciplinary research is primarily concerned with the development and testing of theories to explain social or biological phenomena, while health services research applies the theories and methods that have evolved within these disciplines to investigating problems related to the operation of the medical care delivery system. Further, whereas clinical research is principally concerned with medical-related outcomes and predictors for individual patients, health services research more broadly acknowledges the array of nonmedical (social, economic, and organizational) factors that can affect the operation and outcomes of the medical care system. (See Figure 1.1.)

Definition of policy analysis

Policy analysis has been defined in terms of two principal objectives: (1) the production of information relevant to policymaking, and (2) the development of reasonable arguments translating the information into recommendations for governmental action (Dunn 1981). The distinction drawn here between health services research and policy analysis is that the first objective (the *production* of knowledge) defines the *primary* contributions of health services research and the second (the *application* of knowledge) represents the *primary* contributions of health policy analysis to governmental decision making.

The first objective most directly mirrors the goal of health services research that is concerned with generating knowledge about the implementation and effect of specific health programs and policies. The principal questions and issues being addressed are factual or objective: to document the scope or origins of a problem (proportion of the population and subgroups without insurance coverage) and the probable effectiveness of alternatives for addressing it (cross-national comparisons of alternative systems of financing medical care), for example.

The second objective extends somewhat beyond the role traditionally assumed by health services research. It attempts to justify the relevance of particular types of research, weigh the evidence, and construct a logical case to policymakers regarding the significance of a problem or the utility of specific programs or policies for addressing it. The primary emphases of this objective are normative and persuasive: to provide a logical, well-documented rationale for evaluating the adequacy of existing policies (in providing insurance coverage) and choosing one

Figure 1.1 Comparison of Focus of Health Services Research with Other Types of Research

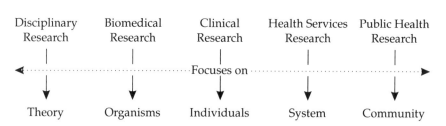

(universal health insurance) alternative over another in the light of competing health policy goals (effectiveness, efficiency, and equity).

The final chapter elaborates how health services research contributes to the research-oriented, as well as the decision-making-oriented, objectives of policy analysis in the context of evaluating major universal health insurance options being debated in U.S. communities and the Congress.

Differences from other types of inquiry

Figure 1.2 contrasts health services research and policy analysis with other types of basic and applied scientific inquiry in terms of the primary research objectives of each. Disciplines (such as economics) provide useful theories (of demand and supply) to explain biological or social phenomena (the operation of consumer and provider behavior in the medical care marketplace). These theories underlie the conduct of health services research to describe and assess the performance of the medical care system (in terms of efficiency, for example). Health program evaluation is concerned with assessing the effect of specific policies and programs (such as state rate-setting systems, physician-reimbursement schemes, or consumer cost-sharing provisions) on a defined policy outcome of interest (cost containment), and applies the concepts and methods of disciplinary research as well as health services research in evaluating these alternatives. The evaluation of the implementation and effect of health care programs (such as neighborhood health centers, hospital-based group practices, or immunization outreach efforts) has been a major component of health services research (Shortell and Richardson 1978). To the extent that such evaluations are directed toward assessing specific governmental policies or programs, they may provide direct input to related health policy analysis efforts. Policy analysis draws upon the fund of knowledge generated by disciplinary and health services research to clarify concerns about current policies (insurance coverage), compare new policy alternatives (universal health insurance proposals), and make recommendations to (national, state, and local) decision makers.

Health services research has historically been criticized for not having been sufficiently involved in the conduct of research that directly informs difficult health policy decisions (Anderson 1991; Choi and Greenberg 1982; Flook and Sanazaro 1973; Institute of Medicine 1979). Recent compilations of the contributions of health services research to health policy and management do, however, clearly indicate that the lines between health services research and policy analysis are more aptly characterized as diffuse, rather than distinct (DeFriese, Ricketts, and Stein 1989; Ginzberg 1991; Shortell and Reinhardt 1992; White 1992).

Figure 1.2 Comparison of Objectives of Health Services Research with Other Types of Inquiry

Type of Inquiry	Objective
Disciplinary Research	To explain biological or social phenomena
	$X \longrightarrow Y$
Health Services Research	To describe and assess the performance of the medical care system
	Structure Process Outcome
	$x \longrightarrow y$
Health Program Evaluation	To evaluate the effect of health policies and programs
	$x_0 \longrightarrow y_0$
	$x_1 \longrightarrow y_1$
	$x_2 \longrightarrow y_2$
	$x_3 \longrightarrow y_3$
Health Policy Analysis	To define problems and compare health policy alternatives
	x_1
	vs.
	$x_2 \longrightarrow y$
	vs.
	x_3

Topics and Applications of Health Services Research

Framework for classifying topics and issues in health services research

Health policy may be viewed as a starting point or motivation for the design and conduct of health services research. (See Figure 1.3.) The access, cost, and quality dilemmas faced by governmental and private institutions at the national, state, and local level in providing and paying for medical care serve as invitations to interested investigators to contribute to the knowledge and expertise needed to address them. The availability of support through government contracts, investigator-initiated studies, and foundation-sponsored research and demonstration projects provides direct incentives for developing research projects, consultative arrangements, or conferences and task forces to study these issues.

The concepts and methods of health services research provide guidance by *describing, analyzing,* and *evaluating* the *structure, process,* and *outcomes* of the medical care system.

Structure refers to the availability, organization, and financing of health care programs and the characteristics of the populations to be served by them. *Process* encompasses the transactions between patients

Figure 1.3   Framework for Classifying Topics and Issues in Health Services Research

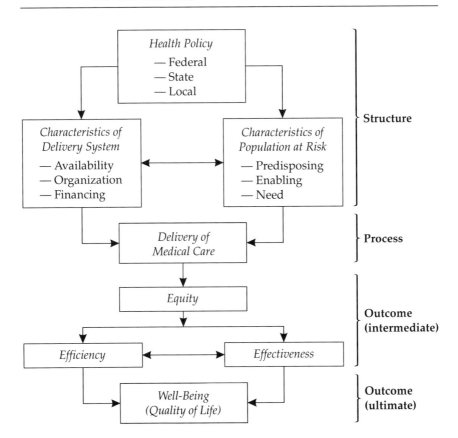

and providers in the course of actual care delivery. Equity, efficiency, and effectiveness may be viewed as intermediate *outcomes* of the medical care delivery process that is ultimately concerned with enhancing the population's health and well-being.

Health services research provides basic descriptive data on the organization and operation of the medical care system (number and distribution of providers, percentage of population uninsured, distribution of medical conditions in the population). It also analyzes likely relationships between and among components—reflected in the arrows in Figure 1.3—examining the impact of health policy on the delivery system and the populations affected by these initiatives, the influence of the characteristics of the delivery system on equity, and the interaction of the efficiency and effectiveness objectives, for example. This model assumes that equity of access to the system, reflected in who gains entry and how often patients use services, has a direct impact on the efficiency and effectiveness of the care that is delivered, as well as ultimately on the quality of life of the population it was intended to serve.

Macro versus micro levels of analysis

The structure, process, and outcomes of medical care can be studied at either the micro (individual patient-provider or institutional) level or the macro (system or community) level. Chapters 2 through 7 examine the performance of the system in terms of effectiveness, efficiency, and equity at both the micro and macro levels.

An exclusive focus on one level of analysis may fail to acknowledge the existence or consequences of the other. Commitments to developing medical technologies or procedures to optimize individual patient outcomes may fail to consider whether these are the best investments to enhance the health and well-being of the population as a whole. On the other hand, a macro-level look at *aggregate* indicators of health status (death rates due to heart disease) and measures of system performance (rates of untreated hypertension) may fail to reveal fully the underlying role that personal lifestyle practices (smoking) and attitudes (toward regular physical activity) play in affecting *individuals'* health status.

Different images of effectiveness emerge when viewed through macro-level lenses focusing on changes in the *population's* health, compared to a micro-level look at outcomes for individual *patients*. The production efficiency of individual health care providers does not of necessity lead to allocative efficiency in the medical care marketplace. Yardsticks of fairness may be applied in assessing the extent to which *either* individual institutions (hospitals or clinics) *or* the delivery system as a whole measure up in terms of the equity objective.

The discussion in the chapters that follow offers additional insights on the performance of the medical care system that may be uniquely illuminated (as well as left out) by a singular focus on either the macro- *or* micro-level point of view.

A Historical Overview of the Contributions of Health Services Research to Health Policy

Health services research is a relatively new field of inquiry, though its origins may be traced to the early 1900s in the United States. Selected historical contributions of health services research to the formulation of health policy are highlighted here. (For more detail, see Anderson 1990 and Flook and Sanazaro 1973.)

The Flexner report, based on a comprehensive study of medical schools in the U.S. and Canada, was published in 1910. This report led to a major reorganization of medical education in the United States.

The Committee on the Costs of Medical Care (CCMC) was established in 1927. That prestigious 42-member committee played a major role in the design and conduct of research on the utilization and costs of care and the inequities of access that existed among income groups. The committee published 28 reports, including a series of recommendations that affected and continue to affect how medical care is organized and delivered in the United States (discussed further in Chapter 6).

In 1935–36, the Public Health Service conducted a National Health Survey and a Business Census of Hospitals to provide basic data on the health and health care needs of the population and the financial structure of U.S. hospitals. An outgrowth of this early research was the development of the concept of health service areas for general hospitals and health centers. In 1944, the American Hospital Association (AHA) established its Commission on Hospital Care that provided the first complete inventory of the nation's hospitals. This and the earlier Business Census identified a need for more general hospital beds, especially in rural areas, that in 1946 resulted in the passage of the Hill-Burton Act, authorizing a massive, nationwide hospital survey and construction program.

The Commission on Chronic Illness, established in 1949 under the auspices of the AHA, the American Medical Association (AMA), the American Public Health Association (APHA), and the American Public Welfare Association (APWA), carried out a number of studies dealing with the community prevalence and prevention of chronic illness, long-term care, and home care. The AHA Commission on Financing, established in 1951, attempted to address many of the issues related to the financing of hospital care (the factors affecting cost, prepayment, and financing care for nonwage and low-income groups) that had not been dealt with directly by the earlier (1944) AHA Commission on Hospital Care. The research carried out by these major commissions contributed to early deliberations concerning the appropriate role of government in health care, as in President Truman's Commission on the Health Care Needs of the Nation, as well as to the development of survey research and statistical and economic analysis methodologies that provide the foundation for contemporary health services research.

The U.S. Department of Health, Education, and Welfare (DHEW) was established in 1953. The National Health Survey Act, which provided authorization for the major data-gathering efforts of the National Center for Health Statistics (NCHS), was passed in 1956. The research undertaken under the auspices of these agencies documented continuing inequities in health and health care on the part of the poor and the elderly in particular, identified over 20 years earlier by the Committee on the Costs of Medical Care. The evidence of these persistent disparities provided an empirical foundation for the passage of the Medicaid and Medicare legislation in 1965 to extend federally subsidized coverage to these groups.

The lead federal agency for support of formal health services research activities, the National Center for Health Services Research and Development (NCHSRD), was established in 1968. During the intervening period, a number of other federal agencies (including the Veterans Administration, Health Care Financing Administration, National Institute of Mental Health, and National Institute of Aging, among others) as well as private foundations (the Robert Wood Johnson Foundation, the Commonwealth Fund, and the Pew Foundation, for example) assumed a greater role in supporting the design and conduct of health services research activities. The first national meeting of the Association for Health Services Research (AHSR) and the Foundation for Health Services Research (FHSR) was held in Chicago in June 1984. In 1989, the National Center for Health Services Research received a substantial boost in funding for patient outcomes and medical effectiveness research as a result of major outcomes research bills introduced by Congress, and the agency itself was subsequently renamed the Agency for Health Care Policy and Research (AHCPR) to reflect its more policy-oriented focus.

Health services research is increasingly making contributions to the design and evaluation of health policies and programs at the federal, state, and local level—such as Medicaid and Medicare payment systems, resource-based relative value methods of reimbursing physicians, and clinical practice guidelines, among others (Brown 1991).

In the chapters that follow, the contributions of health services research, supported by various agencies and organizations, to clarifying and evaluating the health policy objectives of effectiveness, efficiency, and equity are examined.

Overview of the U.S. Medical Care System

The discussion that follows describes trends in the structure, process, and outcomes of the U.S. medical care system as they relate to effectiveness, efficiency, and equity. Data will be presented on the health problems of the population that require medical care services, the availability of resources to meet those needs, the organizational and financial structure of the system, who uses it, and how much it costs. The majority of the data are based on *Health, United States, 1991* (NCHS 1992), a publication of the National Center for Health Statistics.

Characteristics of the population at risk

Predictors and indicators of the health status of the population may be considered as measures of both the need for and the outcomes of medical care. These include lifestyle and risk factors (such as cholesterol levels and cigarette smoking), incidence and prevalence of disease (in general, as well as for specific diseases such as acquired immune deficiency syndrome and hypertension), morbidity reflected in limitation of daily activity, mortality (both general and specific, such as infant mortality), and life expectancy.

Selected lifestyle and risk factors

Coronary heart disease is both the most expensive disease and the most frequent cause of death overall in the United States. The known lifestyle risk factors for developing coronary heart disease include, among others, high serum cholesterol levels and cigarette smoking. The levels of these risk factors in the population are indicators of a major potential burden on the medical care system. Overall, 25 percent of the U.S. population have high serum cholesterol levels (defined as greater than 240 mg) or currently smoke.

A somewhat higher percentage of females (29.2 percent) than males (26.0 percent) and whites (28.0 percent) than blacks (26.2 percent) have high serum cholesterol levels (NCHS 1992, 213). Furthermore, the percentage of the population with high serum cholesterol increases substantially with age, with over 40 percent of those 45 or older having levels above the desired maximum. Since 1960, the proportion of the population with elevated cholesterol has declined in all groups except among black males. Whether this decline is the result of lifestyle changes or medical care is unclear.

While about 25 percent of the adult population currently smoke cigarettes, 35 percent of black males do so (NCHS 1992, 204). Overall, a higher proportion of males (28.3 percent) than females (23.2 percent) are likely to smoke. There are no appreciable differences between the smoking rates of white and black females. Current rates also show substantial declines for all groups from a decade ago.

Incidence and prevalence of disease

Acute conditions reported in the National Health Interview Survey include those that resulted in medical attention or restriction of daily activity. During 1990, Americans experienced two acute conditions on average (NCHS 1992, 201). There is a substantial, inverse relationship between age and the number of acute conditions. In 1990, children under 5 averaged almost four episodes per year and adults 45 years of age and older averaged only one.

However, the prevalence of hypertension, a chronic disease leading to both heart attacks and strokes, demonstrates a direct relationship with age. While the overall prevalence of hypertension is 40 percent in adults, it increases from 16 percent in adults aged 20 to 24 to almost 70 percent in adults over 65 (NCHS 1992, 212). Furthermore, the prevalence of hypertension shows a striking disparity by race, with 50 percent of both black males and females 20 to 74 years of age reporting elevated blood pressure. By contrast, somewhat less than 45 percent of white males and fewer than 35 percent of white females 20 to 74 report having been diagnosed with hypertension. In all groups except the black population, the prevalence of hypertension has been increasing since 1960.

Acquired immune deficiency syndrome (AIDS), however, has put the greatest new demand on the medical care delivery system. The number of new cases reported annually in the United States has risen from 4,000 in 1984 to over 30,000 in recent years. In the United States, AIDS has predominantly been a disease of younger males, with the number of cases being almost seven times as great as for females. There are also striking racial differences in the distribution of AIDS, with 59 percent of the male cases being white and 56 percent of the female and child cases being black (NCHS 1992, 188).

Morbidity

The functional effect of chronic diseases is reflected in the limitation of usual or major activities, assessed by self-reports in the National Health Interview Survey. For 1990, 13 percent of the population reported having some limitation, but only 4 percent of the population reported limitation severe enough to make them unable to carry on their major activity

(NCHS 1992, 200). Males, blacks, and persons with low incomes reported higher-than-average levels of activity limitation. Furthermore, limitation of activity increases directly with age.

Mortality

By category, by numbers, and by age-adjusted death rate, the major cause of death in the United States is diseases of the heart, of which the major subcategory is ischemic heart disease (heart attack). In 1989, 733,000 people died of heart disease (NCHS 1992, 158). Malignant neoplasms (cancer) were second with almost 500,000 deaths, cerebrovascular diseases (principally strokes) were third, accidents fourth, and chronic obstructive lung disease fifth. For all causes together and for each of these causes *except for malignant neoplasms*, for which the rates have stayed level, there has been a slow but steady decline in age-adjusted death rates since the 1950s (NCHS 1992, 156).

Infant mortality rates have also been declining, but significant racial differences persist. Overall, the provisional rate for 1990 was 9.1 deaths per 1,000 live births, 8.2 for white infants and more than twice that rate (17.7) for black infants (NCHS 1992, 141). From 1960 to the present, the black infant mortality has been approximately twice that of whites.

Life expectancy

Life expectancy is a product of death rates and associated risk factors and morbidity. Average life expectancy in the United States has shown a slow but steady increase over time. In 1990, life expectancy for both sexes and all races combined was 75.4 years overall, but it differed by gender and race. White females had the longest life expectancy at 79.3 years, then black females at 74.5 years, white males at 72.6 years, and black males at 66.0 years (NCHS 1992, 140).

Characteristics of the delivery system

The discussion that follows highlights the availability, organization, and financing of the U.S. medical care system and the major changes that have taken place over the past three decades, with a particular focus on physician personnel, hospital facilities, and managed care organizations (see Figure 1.3). Physicians are the primary decision makers regarding the use of health care services, while hospitals absorb the most resources of any major sector. Managed care organizations, which attempt to integrate the delivery and financing functions of medical care, are a growing component of the health services delivery system in the United States.

Availability

In 1960, a worsening physician shortage was perceived to exist in the U.S. There were 259,400 active physicians at that time, or 14 per 10,000 population. Federal and state governments greatly expanded investment in medical schools, which grew from 86 in number in 1960 to 127 in 1982. The annual number of medical graduates increased from 7,081 to 15,985 during the same time period. By the year 2000, there are expected to be 721,600 active physicians in the U.S. and a physician-to-population ratio of 26.9 per 10,000 population (NCHS 1992, 245, 251), which has now triggered concerns about a burgeoning physician surplus (Reinhardt 1991).

The hospital industry has also undergone tremendous changes during the past 30 years. There has been rapid advancement in medical technology, an expansion in outpatient services, a growth in multihospital systems, the emergence of increased competition among hospitals and between hospitals and other providers, and a fundamental change in the Medicare payment system that supplies about half of hospital revenue in the United States. The shift has been from a retrospective reimbursement system to the current prospective payment system (PPS) based on diagnosis-related groups (DRGs).

In 1989, there were 5,808 short-stay hospitals in the United States, 31 percent governmental (mostly local), 56 percent nongovernmental not-for-profit, and 13 percent for-profit. These short-stay hospitals represented a total of 1.01 million beds, with state governmental and nongovernmental, nonprofit hospitals accounting for a somewhat disproportionate share of the beds. While for-profit hospitals control only 10 percent of the beds, this is double their share of the market (5 percent) in 1960 (NCHS 1992, 255).

Community hospital beds per 1,000 population increased from 3.6 in 1960 to 3.8 in 1989, after having risen to 4.5 in 1980. Hospital occupancy has declined from 76 percent in 1960 to 67 percent in 1989. The major decline preceded the Medicare prospective payment system that was phased in beginning in 1984 (NCHS 1992, 255, 258).

Organization

Thirty percent of nonfederal physicians now work in group practice settings, compared to 10.6 percent in 1965. The mean size of physician groups has increased from 6.6 to 9.6 physicians during the same period. Fifty percent of groups contract with one or more health maintenance organizations (HMOs), and 20 percent do business with HMOs on a referral basis. Fifty-six percent of groups contract with one or more preferred provider organizations (PPOs) (AMA 1990). HMOs are organizations that guarantee delivery of a comprehensive prepaid benefit package to a voluntarily enrolled population through an organized system of care. PPOs are organizations that contract to provide services at a discounted rate under conditions of utilization review in exchange for consumer incentives to utilize the PPO network of physicians and hospitals.

One reaction to PPS and other cost-containment strategies was the development of strategic alliances between hospitals. In the proprietary sector, large hospital corporations began purchasing hospitals in different markets and instituting centralized and standardized management practices to achieve greater efficiency and profits. Nonprofit hospitals began affiliations with hospitals in their region of the country to establish referral patterns, share services, and possibly for protection against the expansion of the proprietary chains. Whereas 30 percent of hospitals were affiliated in 1979, about 45 percent were affiliated in 1987, and if that trend continues, about 80 percent will be affiliated by the year 2,000 (Luke, Begun, and Pointer 1989).

Financing

The predominant form of physician payment remains fee-for-service although, as described above, physician affiliations with capitated systems (HMOs) have greatly expanded since the early 1970s. Until recently, physicians controlled how they were paid and what they could charge. This led to high incomes relative to the average full-time employee and relative to other professionals in the United States. In 1987, U.S. physicians had average annual earnings of $132,300, which was 5.4 times the average wage of U.S. workers (OECD 1991).

Efforts to freeze fees began in earnest in 1984. Analysts judged the traditional payment system to be both inefficient and inequitable. The system overpaid procedural care at the expense of visits and consultations, physicians providing identical services received very different fees, and it was difficult to understand and complex to administer. A new physician payment system, the resource-based relative value scale, was developed in response to these problems (Physician Payment Review Commission 1991). In January 1992, HCFA began the five-year transition to this new Medicare resource-based fee system described in more detail in Chapter 5.

While many states have long been experimenting with hospital rate-setting programs, implementation of Medicare's prospective payment system in 1984 was the cornerstone of a movement to contain hospital costs. Under PPS, hospitals are paid a prospectively determined amount per discharge, rather than on a retrospective reasonable-cost basis. Payment varies by DRG category, with capital costs initially paid for on a reasonable-cost basis. Capital costs are now being folded into the DRG rate. Payment rates are updated annually to reflect changes in a hospital input price index (Russell 1989).

Government and private insurers have increased their roles in financing health care services in the U.S. Around 20 percent of personal health expenditures were paid for out of pocket in 1990, compared to 56 percent in 1960. Private insurance, including primarily Blue Cross and Blue Shield plans, employer self-insurance, independent plans, and commercial insurance companies covered 32 percent of the cost in 1990, compared to 21 percent in 1960. Government programs covered 41 percent (11 percent state and local and 30 percent federal) of the cost in 1990, almost double the proportion covered in 1960 (Levit et al. 1991, 50). Despite the growth in government and private insurance, there are over 35 million uninsured persons, and an equal or greater number without adequate insurance coverage (NCHS 1992, 291).

Managed care systems

Managed care encompasses various forms of health maintenance organizations and preferred provider organizations. HMO plans and enrollment have grown rapidly since the early 1970s. From 1976 to 1991, the number of plans increased from 174 to 553, and enrollment increased from about 6 million to 34 million persons. While this represents strong growth, and HMOs are vigorous competitors of traditional health insurance plans in several metropolitan areas, HMOs enroll only about 13 percent of the U.S. civilian population (NCHS 1992, 293). Recent trends include growth in managed care plans such as PPOs and nontraditional HMOs that allow enrollees to select a non-HMO provider in exchange for a financial penalty. Between January 1990 and July 1991, enrollment in these plans (28.5 million) exceeded enrollment in traditional HMOs (25.3 million). Recently, private employers, the federal Medicare program through major risk contracts, and various state/federal Medicaid programs have also attempted to increase their share of beneficiaries' participation in HMOs (InterStudy 1992).

Utilization of the medical care system

Utilization rates reflect encounters between providers and patients, which take place in ambulatory care facilities (doctors' offices or public health clinics), hospitals, and nursing homes, as well as other settings.

Ambulatory services

In 1990, the civilian noninstitutionalized U.S. population averaged 5.5 physician contacts for the year (NCHS 1992, 219). The number of contacts ranged from 4.7 per person per year for males to 6.1 for females. Whites on average had about 10 percent more contacts, with 5.6 per person per year, compared to 5.1 for blacks. Over time, there has been a gradual increase in the average number of contacts per person per year for all groups. One group in particular appears to have been significantly affected by the passage of Medicare and Medicaid in 1965. In 1964, blacks averaged 3.6 physician contacts per person per year, but by 1975 their mean number of visits had risen to 4.9 (NCHS 1983, 90).

In 1989, Americans averaged 2.1 dental visits per person per year (NCHS 1992, 223). Males and females had about an equal number of visits. Whites however averaged 2.3 visits, while blacks logged only 1.2 visits. Whites showed steady increases in visits to dentists from 1964 onward, but the use rate for blacks has remained relatively unchanged since 1983.

Inpatient services

In 1990, there were 91 discharges from short-stay hospitals per 1,000 population in the United States (NCHS 1992, 224). The number did not differ substantially from the average for whites, but the average for blacks was substantially higher at 112 discharges. Subsequent to the passage of Medicare and Medicaid in 1964, the average declined for whites, but blacks experienced a marked jump in discharges from 84 per 1,000 population in 1964 to 115.2 in 1985.

The other important measure of hospital use, besides admissions and discharges, is the average length of stay in days, which reflects a pattern similar to that of admissions over time. In 1990, the average length of stay was 6.7 days, with no significant departures from this average for whites (NCHS 1992, 225). Prior to Medicare and Medicaid (1964), blacks had the highest average length of stay with 12.7 days, versus about 9.0 days overall. For all groups, the average length of stay has declined over time, but the drop has been most dramatic for blacks— to 7.8 days in 1990.

Procedures indicate a costly dimension of hospital use. Two major types of procedures will be examined: diagnostic and other nonsurgical procedures, and surgical operations. The use of procedures and operations tends to be gender-specific, so utilization rates are reported separately for males and females.

Angiocardiography, visualizing the coronary arteries with contrast material, was the most frequent inpatient diagnostic procedure done in males in 1990, with 6.9 procedures per 1,000 population (NCHS 1992, 233). Computerized axial tomography (CAT) scans and diagnostic ultrasound were second and third at 5.8 and 5.4 procedures, respectively. Cystoscopy (viewing the interior of the urinary tract) was fourth at 2.7

procedures. The use of the first three procedures increased about four-fold over the decade; for cystoscopy, the frequency declined slightly.

For females, the same three procedures topped the list but the order was different: first, diagnostic ultrasound; second, CAT scans; and third, angiocardiography. The rates were 6.2, 4.9, and 3.5 respectively. Diagnostic ultrasound was first in females because of its use in visualizing the fetus in pregnancy. Each of these procedures also showed a four-fold increase over the decade since 1980. The fourth most frequent inpatient diagnostic procedure for females was the radioisotope scan at a rate of 2.1 per 1,000 population.

The predominant surgical operations for males, in order, were cardiac catheterization (5.2 per 1,000 population), prostatectomy (2.8), fracture reduction (2.4), and coronary bypass (2.4) (NCHS 1992, 231). Cardiac catheterization rates more than doubled over the decade, while the frequency for each of the other operations declined slightly.

For females the most frequent operations were delivery-related, with normal delivery most frequent by a three-fold margin (17.3 per 1,000 population) over cesarean section (6.6) and episiotomy (5.5). The other frequent operations in women were hysterectomy at 4.3, oophorectomy (removal of an ovary) at 3.4, tubal ligation at 2.9, and dilatation and curettage (D&C) at 0.8. Cesarean-section rates have increased over 25 percent since 1980, while tubal ligations and D&Cs have declined substantially.

Nursing home services

Perhaps one of the most dramatic effects of Medicaid and Medicare has been the increase in the number of residents in nursing homes and personal care settings. As of 1985, there were 46.2 residents 65 years and over per 1,000 population in such settings (NCHS 1992, 236). Females outnumbered males at 57.9 versus 29.0 per 1,000 population, and whites outnumbered blacks at 47.7 versus 35.0 per 1,000 population. The rates have almost doubled for most groups since the enactment of Medicaid and Medicare in 1964, and they have tripled for blacks.

Expenditures and costs

National health care expenditures (NHE) for the complex and highly technological U.S. medical care enterprise were $666.2 billion in 1990 compared to $27.1 billion in 1960. For the same period, health care expenditures grew from $143 to $2,566 per capita and from 5.3 percent to 12.2 percent of the gross national product (GNP) (Levit et al. 1991, 46).

While all national health care expenditures have grown, the 30-year shift in the distribution of spending for services has been mainly toward nursing home and hospital care and away from drugs and other medical sundries. Hospitals represent the largest sector, with the proportion spent in this area increasing from 34 percent in 1960 to 38 percent in 1990 (NCHS 1992, 268). Cost-containment efforts in the 1980s appear to have restrained the growth in hospital expenditures. Expenditures for physician services have held steady at about 20 percent of national health care expenditures. Nursing home expenditures have increased with the aging of the population and expansion of public programs, from 4 percent of total health expenditures in 1960 to 8 percent in 1990. Though the absolute levels of expenditures have increased, the relative shares for drugs and other medical sundries have declined since 1960.

The growth in personal health care expenditures (that is, spending for the direct provision of care) increased sharply after the passage of Medicare and Medicaid in 1965 and continued a strong upward trend in the 1970s, a period of high general inflation. Growth declined initially in the 1980s in response to cost-containment measures and the decline in general inflation. However, cost increases resumed, with growth at 10.5 percent between 1989 and 1990. The major factors affecting growth in personal health expenditures have been economywide inflation, medical price inflation in excess of general inflation, and the increased use and intensity of services per capita (Levit et al. 1991).

In summary, due to often conflicting attempts to address the twin problems of access to care and increasing costs, physicians, hospitals, insurers, and consumers have faced dramatic changes in the organization and financing of medical care during the past 30 years. All of these new arrangements are part of a new corporate medical enterprise in U.S. health care (Starr 1982).

Payers and policymakers are struggling to formulate policy to address these problems in the context of the uniquely pluralistic American health care system.

The chapters that follow examine the conceptual, methodological, and empirical underpinnings of the effectiveness, efficiency, and equity objectives of the U.S. medical care system. The specific application of health services research to decision making regarding outcomes management, physician payment reform, and universal health insurance is reviewed to illustrate the role of health services research in formulating specific policies or programs to achieve these objectives.

In the final chapter the contributions of health services research to policy analysis are demonstrated in comparing alternative universal health insurance options using criteria derived from the effectiveness, efficiency, and equity concepts.

Note

1. More generally, we are concerned about allocating resources among all possible goods and services to achieve maximum social welfare (or well-being).

References

American Medical Association. 1990. *Medical Group Practice in the United States.* Chicago: American Medical Association.

Anderson, O. W. 1991. *The Evolution of Health Services Research: Personal Reflections on Applied Social Science.* San Francisco: Jossey-Bass.

———. 1990. *Health Services as a Growth Enterprise in the United States since 1875.* 2nd ed. Ann Arbor: Health Administration Press.

Brown, L. D. 1991. "Knowledge and Power: Health Services Research as a Political Resource." In *Health Services Research: Key to Health Policy*, edited by E. Ginzberg. Cambridge, MA: Harvard University Press.

Choi, T., and J. N. Greenberg. 1982. *Social Science Approaches to Health Services Research.* Ann Arbor: Health Administration Press.

DeFriese, G. H., T. C. Ricketts, III, and J. S. Stein, eds. 1989. *Methodological Advances in Health Services Research.* Ann Arbor: Health Administration Press.

Dunn, W. N. 1981. *Public Policy Analysis.* Englewood Cliffs, NJ: Prentice-Hall.

Flook, E. E., and P. J. Sanazaro, eds. 1973. *Health Services Research and R&D in Perspective.* Ann Arbor: Health Administration Press.

Ginzberg, E., ed. 1991. *Health Services Research: Key to Health Policy.* Cambridge, MA: Harvard University Press.

Institute of Medicine. 1979. *Report on Health Services Research.* Washington, DC: National Academy of Sciences.

InterStudy. 1992. *1991 Managed Care Firms.* Excelsior, MN: InterStudy.

Levit, K. R., H. C. Lazenby, C. A. Cowan, and S. W. Letsch. 1991. "National Health Expenditures 1990." *Health Care Financing Review* 13 (1): 29–54.

Luke, R. D., J. W. Begun, and D. D. Pointer. 1989. "Quasi-firms: Strategic Interorganizational Forms in the Health Care Industry." *Academy of Management Review* 14 (1): 9–19.

National Center for Health Statistics. 1983. *Health, United States, 1982.* DHHS Pub. No. PHS 83-1232. Washington, DC: U.S. Government Printing Office.

———. 1992. *Health, United States, 1991.* DHHS Pub. No. PHS 92-1232. Washington, DC: U.S. Government Printing Office.

OECD Health Data: A Software Package for the International Comparison of Health Care Systems. 1991. Ver. 1.01. Paris: Organization for Economic Co-operation and Development.

Physician Payment Review Commission. 1991. *Annual Report to Congress, 1991.* Washington, DC: Physician Payment Review Commission.

Reinhardt, U. E. 1991. "Health Manpower Forecasting: The Case of Physician Supply." In *Health Services Research: Key to Health Policy*, edited by E. Ginzberg. Cambridge, MA: Harvard University Press.

Russell, L. B. 1989. *Medicare's New Hospital Payment System: Is It Working?* Washington, DC: Brookings Institution.

Shortell, S. M., and U. E. Reinhardt, eds. 1992. *Improving Health Policy and Management: Nine Critical Research Issues for the 1990s.* Ann Arbor: Health Administration Press.

Shortell, S. M., and W. C. Richardson. 1978. *Health Program Evaluation.* St. Louis: C. V. Mosby.

Starr, P. 1982. *The Social Transformation of American Medicine.* New York: Basic Books.

White, K. L. 1992. *Health Services Research: An Anthology.* Scientific Publication No. 534. Washington, DC: Pan American Health Organization, Pan American Sanitary Bureau, Regional Office of the World Health Organization.

Chapter 2

Effectiveness: Concepts and Methods

Does medical care do any good? While that question has been asked often, it is deceptively simple and misleading. Implicit in it are two more fundamental questions: (1) what are the contributions of medical care to the health of the population; and (2) can the clinical effectiveness of medical care be improved? Both of these questions concern effectiveness—the actual achieved benefits of medical care. The purpose of this chapter is to define the concept of effectiveness of medical care and to examine the key methods for assessing effectiveness.

A place to begin in addressing the first question is to examine how the mortality experience of the population has changed over time in the United States and the contributions of medical care to any improvements observed. Mortality from all major infectious diseases has declined over this century in the United States. Over a 75-year period, the standardized mortality rate from tuberculosis fell from over 200 deaths per 100,000 population to less than 10. Deaths from pneumonia dropped from over 150 deaths per 100,000 population to less than 25. Significant declines in mortality from diphtheria and typhoid fever, as well as for other infectious diseases, occurred also during the period from 1900 to 1973 and have continued to the present (McKinlay and McKinlay 1977).

Infant mortality rates followed a similar and related pattern with a rapid decline from high levels of 60 deaths per 1,000 live births in 1930 to 29.2 by 1950. The decline of 4.3 percent per year slowed to 2.0 percent per year by 1950 but resumed a sharp decline of about 5 percent per year in 1970 when the rate was 20 deaths per 1,000 live births. By 1990 the provisional rate had reached 9.1. For blacks the rates have been higher throughout the century, but the pattern is similar. It was almost

100 deaths per 1,000 live births in 1930, 43.9 in 1950, 32.2 in 1970, and 17.7 in 1989 (NCHS 1992, 141).

In the 1940s, however, the Public Health Service published a set of analyses (Moriyama and Gover 1948; Woolsey and Moriyama 1948) that documented not only the decline in acute infectious disease mortality but a significant and rapid increase in mortality from chronic diseases, particularly coronary heart disease. Adjusted for the changing age distribution of the population, the data revealed that coronary heart disease mortality increased from a modest level of 168 deaths per 100,000 population in 1900 to 339 by 1940. The proportion of mortality accounted for by heart disease deaths during the same period had risen from 8 percent to 27 percent. The inexorable increase was followed by a leveling of heart disease mortality, which gave way at first to an imperceptible decline and ultimately to a significant and steady decline in coronary heart disease mortality, which has continued to this day.

During the same time period, life expectancy, which reflects not only declining rates of mortality but also delayed mortality, has been steadily increasing for both men and women and for blacks and whites. At the beginning of the century, life expectancy for white males was only 47 years, but by 1960 it had reached 67 years. By 1980 it was 70 years, and in 1990 was 73 years. White female life expectancy at the turn of the century was 49 years. It has always been higher than white male life expectancy but has followed a similar pattern, reaching a current level of 79 years. Similar patterns but lower levels have consistently existed for black males and females, at 66 years and 75 years in 1990, respectively (NCHS 1992, 140).

The near elimination of acute infectious disease mortality, the significant decline in infant mortality, the sharp reductions in the major causes of death (except for cancer mortality, which has stayed level), and the resulting increase in life expectancy appeared to herald a new era of accomplishments in the health care arena. These successes, however, were followed not by a new generation growing up free of disease but by a new and frightening infectious disease epidemic. In a little over a decade, acquired immune deficiency syndrome has emerged as the ninth major cause of death overall and the second leading cause of death for men aged 25 to 44 in the United States. Health, as the eradication of all diseases, infectious or otherwise, does indeed seem to be a "mirage" as Rene Dubos (1959) has suggested.

There is no question, then, that the health of the population in the United States has improved substantially over this century as judged by mortality and life expectancy figures. But are these improvements in fact attributable to medical care or to some other factor or set of factors? There are differing opinions on the answer to this question, and three viewpoints representative of the range of opinion are presented here, setting the stage for a discussion of the effectiveness of medical care.

Thomas McKeown, Ivan Illich, and Rick Carlson, writing in the 1970s, joined what might be called a nihilistic chorus proclaiming repeatedly that whatever improvements there were in the health of the population were in fact due to forces other than medical care. Illich and Carlson believed medical care had, by the early 1970s, become a major *cause* of death and disability.

Illich (1975), perhaps the most radical of these analysts, argued in his book, *Medical Nemesis,* that not only is medicine of limited effectiveness, but that since the 1950s medicine has had the potential to cause as much harm as good. Carlson (1975) echoed a similar thought in his book, *The End of Medicine,* arguing that even the limited effectiveness of medical care would decline. He further asserted, as had others, that social and environmental factors contribute more to improving the health of the population than medical care. McKeown (1976), drawing upon Western mortality patterns over nearly a century, argued that the reductions in mortality were due mainly to improvements in nutrition and hygiene, not to medical care.

Less nihilism was reflected in such writings as Victor Fuchs's book, *Who Shall Live?* (1974), which did not dispute the contributions of medical care but argued that its marginal contributions were small. In other words, while great gains had been achieved in the past, further increments in the investment in medical care were not likely to bring substantial improvements in the health of the population. Fuchs and others like him—for example, Lester Breslow (Berkman and Breslow 1983) and John Knowles (1977)—advocated nonmedical interventions such as lifestyle change.

Milio (1983) went further in her analysis. She presented evidence on the limited effectiveness of medical care in addressing both the acute and chronic health problems of the population. Instead of individual behavior change she advocated large-scale social change to mitigate the destructive influences of modern life. Evans and Stoddart (1990) additionally argued that spending great sums of wealth on marginally effective medical care reduces savings, investment, and prosperity and may ultimately have a negative effect on health as well. They pointed to Japan as the society that has achieved the greatest improvements in all these economic measures during the past 40 years and now demonstrates the best showing on measures of the health of the population. A major policy implication, in their view, is that stopping or drastically slowing the growth in medical care spending is the way to improve health.

A third perspective, typified by Avedis Donabedian, John Williamson, Robert Brook, and John Wennberg, has accepted the evidence of medical care's current limits, but has, instead of advocating social and behavioral change, addressed the question of whether the benefits of medical care can be improved. Their answer to this question is a resounding, "Yes," and they believe that health services research, particularly in the form of what is now called outcomes research, can lead to these improvements. Donabedian (1966) provided a framework for this line of research, arguing that it was time to cease worrying about how to measure quality of medical care and get on with the determination of the linkages between the structural components, processes, and outcomes of medical care.

Williamson, a pioneer in conceptualizing the field of research related to the outcomes of medical care, contributed substantially to the emphasis on outcomes and methods of study (Williamson, Alexander, and Miller 1968). His book on health accounting (Williamson 1978) advocated an accounting approach to quality improvement. He argued for a quality assurance system analogous to the process of financial accounting. In 1991, he called for a new approach to improving the quality of medical care, an outcomes framework for improving quality management, and labeled it LARGE QA (quality assurance) (Williamson, Moore, and Sanazaro 1991).

Brook, writing with Lohr (1985), called for an epidemiology of medical care, meaning the systematic investigation of the linkages between the component parts of medical care and patients' health outcomes. This is an agenda that Brook has pursued through a career of empirical studies, beginning with his doctoral dissertation comparing five methods of medical care peer review (Brook 1974).

Wennberg, based on the documentation and investigation of the geographic variations in use of medical care (Wennberg and Gittelsohn 1973), has led a new group of researchers into what he is calling clinical evaluation science (Wennberg 1990). This new science encompasses the systematic investigation of what procedures in medical care contribute to better outcomes for individual patients and how those procedures can be disseminated and encouraged.

The policy outcome of all these arguments has been the enactment of legislation to study the determinants of better medical care outcomes and to seek to improve them. Ellwood (1988) labeled, described, and defined this field of activity as outcomes management, and Relman (1988) heralded its beginning as the Era of Accountability. The harbingers of this era were the releases of hospital mortality statistics by the Health Care Financing Administration (HCFA) for 1984 and 1986 (Health Care Financing Administration 1986, 1987). These two reports documented and made public the tremendous variation in mortality outcomes experienced by patients treated in different hospitals. At the same point in time the Joint Commission on Accreditation of Healthcare Organizations (JCAHO) adopted its Agenda for Change, which called for the establishment of clinical indicators (including outcomes), review of hospital care, and the input of these data into a national data base (O'Leary 1987).

Two bills to develop medical practice guidelines and improve the effectiveness of medical care were introduced in the U.S. Congress in 1989. The result was the passage of PL 101-239, which established the Agency for Health Care Policy and Research, formerly the National Center for Health Services Research. The agency's agenda is to investigate variations in medical practice as they relate to outcomes, and to develop and disseminate practice guidelines to improve patient care.

This chapter and the next address the questions of how medical care contributes to improving health and whether its effectiveness can be enhanced. In this chapter, a conceptual framework for effectiveness research is described. Following that description and the distinguishing of two complementary definitions of effectiveness, key methods of effectiveness research are presented.

Chapter 3 reviews the evidence from effectiveness research as it relates to the two principal questions posed at the beginning of this chapter. Finally, Chapter 3 presents and discusses a current application of effectiveness research to health policy—the outcomes assessment activities currently being funded by the Agency for Health Care Policy and Research.

Conceptual Framework and Definitions

The major conceptual frameworks that guide effectiveness research derive from the work of Donabedian, Brook, and Wennberg. Donabedian (1966) first offered the categorization of medical care in terms of structure, process, and outcomes for the purpose of determining what aspects might be indicators of quality. Since that time, this categorization and the implied linkage among these components have become the basics for studying the effectiveness of medical care and its determinants. These relationships are captured in the summary framework shown at the top of Table 2.1.

The conceptualization in Table 2.1 illustrates that structure, process, and outcome are linked conceptually in a research paradigm that assumes that structural elements of medical care influence what is and is not done in the medical care process, as well as how well it is done, and that this process in turn influences the outcome, health, which people experience as a result of their encounters with the medical care process.

Table 2.1 Summary Framework and Definitions: Effectiveness

STRUCTURE ⟶	PROCESS ⟶	OUTCOMES
Quantity Efficacy	Variations in Use — Quantity — Quality — Appropriateness	Effectiveness — Mortality — Clinical outcomes — Functional
Quantity The number of physicians, nurses, and other providers as well as the quantity of monetary resources.	**Variations in Use** "Different observed levels of per capita consumption of a service, especially hospital care, office visits, drugs, and specific procedures" (Brook and Lohr 1985).	**Effectiveness** "Achieved benefit" (Williamson 1978). "*Does it work?*" "Does the maneuver, procedure, or service do more good than harm to those people to whom it is offered?" (Sackett 1980).
Efficacy "Maximum *achievable* benefit" (Williamson 1978). "*Can it work?*" "Does the health maneuver, procedure, or service do more good than harm to people who fully comply with the associated recommendations or treatment?" (Sackett 1980). The ability of "a particular medical action [to alter] the natural history of a particular disease for the better," under ideal conditions (adapted from Cochrane 1971).	**Quality** "A judgment concerning the process of care, based on the extent to which that care contributes to valued outcomes" (Donabedian 1982). "That component of the difference between efficacy and effectiveness that can be attributed to care providers, taking account of the environment in which they work" (Brook and Lohr 1985). **Appropriateness** "The extent to which available knowledge and techniques are used or misused in the management of illness and health" (Donabedian 1973).	The ability of "a particular medical action [to alter] the natural history of a particular disease for the better," under actual conditions of practice and use (adapted from Cochrane 1971).

Definitions

An explanation of the terms in this framework is required. The lower half of Table 2.1 provides detailed examples of several illustrative definitions for each of these terms, while the discussion that follows summarizes the key idea implicit in each of them. *Efficacy* is concerned with the benefits achievable from a therapy or an intervention under ideal conditions, such as are found in a randomized clinical trial (Brook and Lohr 1985; Cochrane 1971; Sackett 1980; Williamson 1978). *Variations in use* relate to the quantity, or what is more commonly referred to as utilization, of medical care services and procedures (Brook and Lohr 1985). It includes the frequency, or volume, of procedures done.

Quality is an attribute of the medical care process having to do with both whether the right thing is done and whether it is done well (Brook and Lohr 1985; Donabedian 1980, 1988). *Quality assessment* thus deals with evaluating this aspect of the process of medical care. *Appropriateness* is the subset of quality that is concerned with determining whether the right thing was done for the patient. *Effectiveness* concerns the results achieved in the actual practice of medical care with typical patients and providers, as contrasted to efficacy which is assessed by the benefits achieved under ideal conditions (Brook and Lohr 1985; Cochrane 1971; Sackett 1980; Williamson 1978). Quality is that part of the gap between efficacy, what is achievable, and effectiveness, what is achieved, which can reasonably be attributed to medical care itself. *Outcomes assessment* addresses the issue of effectiveness by examining the linkages between structures and medical care processes on the one hand, and valued outcomes on the other (Ellwood 1988; Wennberg 1984).

Toward an epidemiology of medical care

That structures influence medical care processes, and that processes influence outcomes, are researchable hypotheses. It is the task of health services research and specifically that part of health services research focused on effectiveness to examine these linkages. Ultimately, this research can provide the basis for health policy decisions concerning which medical care resources and services should receive financial coverage.

Effectiveness research, however, reflects two seemingly competing, but probably complementary, definitions of effectiveness. One is a population perspective, which might be called the macro-level view of the medical care system and its interactions with the social and political systems in achieving improvements in the health of the population. It is represented in the conceptual work of Milio (1983) and can be characterized as the *epidemiology of health*. It includes in its purview both patients who have reached medical care and people in the general population who may not be using medical care. Effectiveness research with this focus is directed at answering the first of the questions introduced at the beginning of this chapter: namely, what are the contributions of medical care to the health of the population?

The second is a clinical perspective, which might be called the micro-level view of medical care, focused on the interactions of patients and providers in the medical care system and the resulting clinical improvement or health benefits achieved by patients. The focus is on the interactions of medical care structures and processes in achieving improvements in the health of patients. It is represented in the work of Donabedian, Wennberg, who has even labeled this area "clinical evaluation science," and Brook and Lohr (1985), who have called for an *epidemiology of medical care*. Effectiveness research with this focus is directed at answering the second of the questions introduced at the beginning of this chapter: namely, can the clinical effectiveness of medical care be improved?

Figure 2.1 discloses the difference in these two views. The population view attends to the health of the population as a whole and to all of the factors contributing to it. The clinical view tends to treat the magnitude of the problem as being related only to that proportion of the population utilizing medical care, and assumes that medical care is the primary means of improving health.

Figure 2.1   Factors Contributing to Public Health

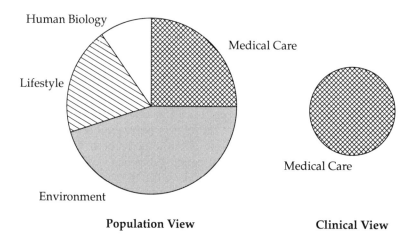

The research related to each of these views mirrors their differing perspectives. The epidemiology of health focuses on the benefits from medical care and other factors to the health of the *population*. The epidemiology of medical care, or clinical evaluation science, delineates the benefits from medical care for *patients*. Two quantitative examples which illustrate these differing views follow.

Assessing population effectiveness

Milio, in discussing the benefits and limitations of primary medical care, developed a framework for assessing effectiveness that links data on the prevalence of the problem in the population, utilization rates, efficacy of recommended treatment procedures, and patient compliance to effectiveness for acute and chronic problems brought to primary care (Milio 1983). Table 2.2 demonstrates her approach for the medical treatment of hypertension. By her definition, the effectiveness of medical care is evaluated in terms of the proportion of the population with a particular problem, for example hypertension, who are benefited by medical care. As can be seen from this illustration, she defines effectiveness as being the product of the percentage of problems brought to primary care (81 percent), the percentage prescribed a specified treatment (27 percent for drug therapy), the efficacy of the prescribed treatment (43 percent), and the patient compliance with that therapy (30 percent). The product of these estimates yields 2.8 percent as the percentage of the prevalence of hypertension improved by drug therapy alone. When these numbers are combined with similar analyses for the effectiveness of weight control and not smoking, Milio derives an overall effectiveness figure of 11.8 percent as primary medical care's contribution to reducing hypertension in the population. In this approach, she not only takes account of the provider side but also includes utilization of medical care and compliance by patients. Using this same approach for a number of acute and chronic medical conditions, she estimates primary medical care's overall effectiveness in addressing the health problems of the population to be 25 percent. This estimate of medical care effectiveness is the basis for the proportion reflected in Figure 2.1.

Assessing clinical effectiveness

Williamson (1978) offers a contrasting view. Williamson defines clinical effectiveness as the ratio of benefit achieved in actual practice to maximum achievable benefit, often from a clinical trial (see Table 2.3). Using hypertension again as the example, and using data from the Veterans Administration (VA) study (VA Cooperative Study Group 1970) of efficacy and the Hypertension Detection and Follow-up Program (HDFP

Table 2.2   A Population Method of Effectiveness Estimation Using
Hypertension as the Example

Use	×	Specific Care	×	Efficacy	×	Compliance	=	Effectiveness
81%	×	27%	×	43% drugs	×	30%	=	2.8%
81%	×	34%	×	100% not smoking	×	32%	=	8.8%
81%	×	38%	×	1.5% weight control	×	52%	=	0.2%
Net								11.8%

Source: Adapted, with the permission of the author, from N. Milio, *Primary Care and the Public's Health* (Lexington, MA: Lexington Books, 1983), 55.

1979) (both presented in the evidence section of the next chapter), Williamson's approach yields an estimate of primary medical care's effectiveness as 62 percent. Specifically, the VA study suggested the maximum conceivable benefit in terms of mortality reduction could be as much as 9.8 percent. The achieved benefit is thus 9.8 percent minus the 7.5 percent mortality level achieved in actual practice, or 2.3 percent. The maximum achievable benefit is 9.8 percent minus the 6.1 percent mortality achieved under ideal conditions, or 3.7 percent. The ratio of these two percentages yields the clinical effectiveness index of 62 percent.

The difference in the two views, the clinical and the population perspectives, leads to widely varying empirical estimates of primary care effectiveness: 62 percent versus 11.8 percent. The next chapter addresses both perspectives, exploring the key methods of effectiveness research and the evidence on effectiveness derived from this research.

Key Methods of Assessing the Effectiveness of Medical Care

The obvious, but oversimplified, question for medical care effectiveness research is, does medical care do any good? The pertinent underlying questions, however, are, what are the contributions of medical care to the health of the population, and can the clinical effectiveness of medical care be improved?

There are basically two levels of analysis and types of studies directed toward these questions. The population perspective described above as the epidemiology of health is aimed at answering the first

Table 2.3   A Clinical Method of Effectiveness Estimation Using Hypertension as the Example

---

The Effectiveness Index

$$\text{Effectiveness} = \frac{\text{Achieved Benefit}}{\text{Maximum Achievable Benefit}}$$

Achieved Benefit

$$\text{Mortality Rate} = \frac{\text{Deaths}}{\text{Persons}} = \frac{368}{4{,}926} = 7.5\%$$

Achieved Benefit =
Maximum Conceivable Reduction − Achieved Mortality Rate

$$= 9.8\% - 7.5\% = 2.3\%$$

Maximum Achievable Benefit

$$\text{Mortality Rate} = \frac{\text{Deaths}}{\text{Persons}} = \frac{301}{4{,}951} = 6.1\%$$

Maximum Achievable Benefit =
Maximum Conceivable Reduction − Achieved Mortality Rate

$$= 9.8\% - 6.1\% = 3.7\%$$

Calculated Effectiveness Index for Hypertension

$$\text{Effectiveness} = \frac{\text{Achieved Benefit}}{\text{Maximum Achievable Benefit}}$$

$$= \frac{2.3\%}{3.7\%} = 62\%$$

Sources: HDFP 1979; VA Cooperative Study Group 1970; Williamson 1978.

underlying question. The clinical perspective described above as the epidemiology of medical care, or clinical evaluation science, is aimed at answering the second.

Table 2.4 outlines the research methodology used to seek answers to these effectiveness questions: the measurement of health status as well as its adjustment for patients' severity of illness (called risk adjustment), the study designs used most often, and the data sources, along with examples of these components. The section that follows discusses effectiveness research methods.

Table 2.4   Key Methods for Effectiveness Research

Methods	Examples
Measurement Variables	
Health status	
Individual measures	
Clinical or physiologic	Blood pressure
Death and disability	
Health-related quality of life	
Generic	Sickness Impact Profile, Medical Outcomes Study, Quality of Well-Being Scale
Disease-specific	Arthritis Impact Measurement Scale
Population-based measures	
Mortality and morbidity	
Disease prevalence and incidence	
Growth and development	
Social and economic productivity	
Risk adjustment	
Subjective	
Objective	
ICD-9-CM-based	Disease Staging, Patient Management Categories
Medical record data–based	Acute Physiology and Chronic Health Evaluation, Computerized Severity Index, MedisGroups
Study Designs	
Randomized clinical trials and social experiments	
Meta-analysis and information synthesis	
Cross-sectional studies	
Decision analysis	
Data Sources	
Population and provider surveys	NCHS National Health Interview Survey
Birth and death registries	U.S. Vital Statistics, World Health Organization
Disease registries	National Cancer Institute Surveillance Epidemiology and End Results
Medical records–based	
Claims data	Medicare Provider Analysis and Review
Hospital discharge data	Commission on Professional and Hospital Activities, Joint Commission on Accreditation of Healthcare Organizations

Measurement variables

Assessing the health of the population requires determining the appropriate measures of health outcomes to use. Both individual and population-based measures of health outcomes have a place in assessing the effectiveness of medical care.

The usefulness of a measure depends, in part, upon the degree to which it meets criteria of reliability, validity, sensitivity, and feasibility. Reliability concerns the reproducibility of the measure under varying conditions of administration. Validity relates to the accuracy of the measure in the sense of its measuring what it is intended to measure. Feasibility refers to the ease with which the scale can be used in various populations. Sensitivity refers to the ability of the measure to detect changes, improvement or deterioration, in the condition of the person as a result of medical care. Sensitivity to medical care variation is particularly important for health outcome measures being used to assess the effectiveness of medical care.

Table 2.5 provides a comparison of several health status measures using these criteria. While these measures are reliable and valid as well as feasible in terms of the ease of getting the information, they differ markedly in their sensitivity to specific medical care interventions. In addition, mortality, a population-based health status measure, has been shown to be much more sensitive to social and demographic variations than to medical care variations (Martini et al. 1977). These individual and population-based health status measures as well as the selected examples listed in Table 2.5 will be discussed next.

Individual health status measures

Individual measures focus on clinical or physiologic outcomes such as blood pressure, on general health status outcomes such as death and disability, and on health-related quality of life measures (refer again to the left-hand column of Table 2.4). Health-related quality of life measures may be of a generic type, applicable across all disease conditions, or of a disease-specific type. Both types are needed in the assessment of the outcomes for medical care, the generic types for comparisons across disease conditions and the disease-specific ones to identify more sensitively the impact of diseases upon people and how treatments affect particular disease conditions. A range of possible health-related quality of life measures is collected in *Measuring Health—A Guide to Rating Scales and Questionnaires* (McDowell and Newell 1987). This book presents, for each of over 100 instruments, a description, copies of the actual questionnaire, information on the reliability and validity of the instrument, and a complete listing of references.

Table 2.5 Comparison of Health Status Measures

Instrument	Reliability	Validity	Feasibility	Sensitivity
Sickness Impact Profile (SIP)	Test-retest 0.90 Internal consistency 0.94	With: —self assessment —physician rating —multiple physiologic measures —other instruments	136 items Self or interview 20–30 minutes	Sensitive to standard medical interventions
Medical Outcomes Study (MOS)	Internal consistencies 0.81–0.88	By comparisons to longer form measures	20 items Self 10 minutes	No information available
Quality of Well-Being Scale (QWB)	Test-retest 0.93 Interrater 0.90	Scale score with —symptoms $r = -0.75$ —problems $r = -0.96$	18 items Interviewer 15 minutes	Sensitive to minor changes
Arthritis Impact Measurement Scale (AIMS)	Reproducibility 0.88 Internal consistency 0.60	Scores with —disease activity $r = 0.61$ —Arthritis Rheumatism Association class $r = 0.66$	45 items Self 15 minutes	Reflects change following treatment
Mortality	High	High	Easily elicited	Modest, more responsive to environment and sociodemographics

Source: McDowell and Newell 1987.

Examples of generic health-related quality of life measures are the Sickness Impact Profile (SIP), the Medical Outcomes Study (MOS) questionnaire, and the Quality of Well-Being Scale (QWB). The SIP (Bergner et al. 1981) and the MOS (Stewart, Hays, and Ware 1988) questionnaires each contain an array of questions related to the effect of disease on physical health, mental health, and social health as well as health perceptions. For these two questionnaires, the scores on each dimension (e.g., physical, mental, social) are separate and presented as a profile. These profiles have been shown to be reliable and valid. They differ in feasibility since the SIP has 136 items and the MOS has only 20 items. The SIP has been shown to be sensitive to standard medical interventions, but the MOS has yet to be tested using this criterion (see Table 2.5).

In response to the current policy demands for a single measure reflecting both the dimensions of health and the utility of various outcomes to patients, instruments such as the Quality of Well-Being (QWB) Scale (Kaplan and Bush 1982) have been developed. For this instrument, an interviewer asks a patient a series of questions about his or her functional level with regard to mobility, physical activity, and social activity. The responses are used to classify a person into one of almost 50 unique functional health states, each of which has been given a normative rating of well-being, ranging between 0 for dead and 1 for perfectly healthy. This allows each health state, regardless of disease condition and person, to be given a well-being rating. This rating can in turn be translated into quality-adjusted life-years (QALYs), and comparisons for policy purposes can be made across diseases, persons, and treatments. More important, such measures go beyond assessing outcomes of medical care in terms of survival only. They bring quality of life into economic decision making regarding which types of care produce the greatest benefits (or utilities) for consumers.

In addition to the generic measures, there are also disease-specific health-related quality of life measures such as the Arthritis Impact Measurement Scale (AIMS) questionnaire (Meenan, Gertman, and Mason 1980). Such questionnaires focus on unique aspects of the disease for which they were developed. They are, as illustrated by the AIMS questionnaire, reliable, valid, feasible, and above all sensitive to the changes following medical treatment (see Table 2.5).

The best health-related quality of life measurement strategy, given the differing levels of sensitivity, is to use a generic instrument, such as the Sickness Impact Profile, supplemented with disease-specific questions or questionnaire (Patrick and Deyo 1989). The generic instrument allows comparisons to be made for economic decisions across diseases, while the disease-specific instrument is more likely to provide sufficient sensitivity to detect small changes in patients' conditions.

Population-based health status measures

Population-based measures (see Table 2.4) include mortality rates, morbidity rates, disease prevalence and incidence rates, growth and development data, and social and economic productivity measures (Hansluwka

1985). Mortality rates can be obtained from U.S. Vital Statistics data as well as from World Health Organization (WHO) data for international comparisons. Morbidity rates can be acquired from NCHS National Health Interview Surveys (NHIS). These surveys are conducted annually on a sample of the U.S. population and yield, among other data, information on limited activity days and restricted activity days. Disease prevalence and incidence data can also be obtained from NHIS data, as well as from other federal sources such as the Centers for Disease Control's *Mortality and Morbidity Weekly Report*. Growth and development measures such as nutritional status and weight for age for this country can be obtained from the Health and Nutrition Examination Surveys also carried out by NCHS. International data of this type can be found in various WHO publications such as the *World Health Statistics Annual*.

Population-based data, as exemplified by mortality (see Table 2.5), while high in reliability, validity, and feasibility, have been repeatedly shown to be insensitive to medical care variation. This suggests that they are useful for addressing the question of medical care's contribution to the health of the population, but they have limited applicability to assessing the clinical effectiveness of medical care.

Risk adjustment

Risk adjustment of patient outcomes, adjustment for patients' severity of illness, is undertaken, and necessary, in effectiveness research to account for the differing beginning severities of patients' presenting complaints. Clearly, patients who differ at admission to a hospital in the severity of their clinical state, and who receive similarly effective treatments, will experience different outcomes. When randomized clinical trials are possible, these differences can be minimized by the random allocation of subjects to experimental and control groups. But under nonexperimental conditions, as with most effectiveness research, these differences, and their potential confounding, should be adjusted for in the analysis.

Two general approaches may be taken in this adjustment. A subjective approach, relying on the informed judgments of experienced clinicians in rating the severity of the patient's illness at entry, may provide a valid assessment of a patient's status, but such an expensive procedure, in terms of the physician's time, is rarely possible. In its place, an objective approach, utilizing clearly identified data related to the patient's clinical state and probable outcome, are used in an algorithm or formula to generate a score characterizing the patient's severity of illness. The risk-adjustment methods in common use, which are described below, take such an objective approach. Risk-adjustment methods do, however, differ in the level of data required to define a patient's severity of illness.

Basic demographic data such as the age and gender of the patient as well as co-morbid conditions were used by Luft, Bunker, and Enthoven (1979) in their study of surgical outcomes and by Dubois and his colleagues (1987) in their study of hospital mortality and quality. These measures are acknowledged to be crude, although the data are readily available.

A somewhat further specification is realized in systems such as the coded version of Disease Staging (DS) and Patient Management Categories (PMCs), which can be constructed with only data from hospital discharge data bases. Specifically, they use information coded according to the *International Classification of Diseases, 9th Revision, Clinical Modification* (ICD-9-CM), from the hospital discharge abstract, to assign severity levels.

The measures with greatest clinical detail—presumably the best measures—are those that require actual medical record–level data for their construction. These include the Acute Physiology and Chronic Health Evaluation (APACHE), the Computerized Severity Index (CSI), and MedisGroups. APACHE was developed for the evaluation of patients in hospital critical care units and uses several physiologic values of the patient generated from laboratory data (Knaus, Draper, and Wagner 1985). It is generic in that it can be applied across diseases for comparisons of severity.

The CSI was developed by Horn and other researchers at Johns Hopkins for the purpose of estimating a hospitalized patient's severity of illness, using information from the total medical record (Horn and Horn 1986). It draws upon information related to the disease stage, complications, co-morbid conditions, dependency on hospital staff, life support, rate of response to therapy, and impairment remaining after treatment. This wide range of information drawn from the entire hospitalization emphasizes that this instrument was developed to reflect resource use and not simply the patient's severity of illness at admission.

MedisGroups has assumed great importance because several states have now mandated it as their risk adjustment measure. The MedisGroups system produces a generic set of severity categories across illnesses, using medical record data processed by a proprietary program (Brewster et al. 1985). It uses what are called "key clinical findings," including laboratory, radiology, pathology, and physical examination data. This information and its coding allow the system to classify patients as to admission severity and to monitor their progress over the hospitalization.

These risk-adjustment methods and severity-of-illness measures can and should be evaluated by the same criteria as health status measures, namely, reliability, validity, feasibility, and sensitivity. Several reviews have summarized the information from the few studies comparing measures in terms of these attributes (Geehr 1989; Hornbrook 1982; Iez-zoni 1990; Thomas and Ashcraft 1991). Basically, the objective methods, because they use factual data and because they are computerized, are both reliable and feasible. Their validity continues to be a question, and they vary in sensitivity, with the systems using only ICD-9-CM data being the least sensitive.

As these reviews show, perhaps the biggest problem with these measures is their use for purposes other than those for which they were initially designed. Several of them were developed to characterize the case mix in an institution for the purposes of determining appropriate resource consumption. As such, they use data from throughout the hospital stay as well as information about procedures done. That is acceptable for case-mix determinations, but when the need is to classify patients at admission, then data from later in the hospitalization may confound the use of the instrument. Furthermore, using other than admission information also confuses severity with the quality of medical care; information generated later may reflect better quality care and the lack of such information may be an indicator of poor quality care. A study that examined this issue for MedisGroups found, for example, that data from the midpoint of the hospital admission provided a better predictor of 30-day mortality than did admission data (Iezzoni, Ash, Coffman, and Moskowitz 1991).

Study designs

Randomized clinical trials

The assessment of efficacy, the determination of the benefits of a partic-ular medical therapy under ideal conditions, involves the randomized clinical trial as the primary method of primary analysis. The hallmark of the randomized clinical trial is random assignment of patients to experimental and control groups, and hence, control of much of the extraneous variation and sources of error. It is a powerful method, but not often feasible because of the expense necessitated by the large sample sizes and the length of time required. Furthermore, ethical issues involved in depriving patients of treatment may also preclude its use. There are, however, several good examples of randomized clinical trials concerning medical interventions, such as propranolol in the treatment of patients with acute myocardial infarction (Beta-Blocker Heart Attack Study Group 1982) and niacin as a preventive of future heart attacks (Canner et al. 1986). Randomized clinical trial designs have also been used to assess the benefits of how medical care is delivered, as in the evaluation of inpatient versus outpatient cardiac catheterization (Block et al. 1988) and day hospital versus inpatient care for cancer patients (Mor et al. 1988). This design has also been used to assess the effects of differing medical care payment plans on use and outcomes (Brook et al. 1983).

Meta-analysis

Because of the difficulties and expense inherent in randomized clinical trials, they must be used selectively. As a result, many important treatment questions cannot be answered. Instead, synthetic methods such as meta-analysis are used in the determination of efficacy. Meta-analysis involves quantitatively and statistically combining the results of several randomized clinical trials to estimate the results of therapy, when no one of the single trials may be sufficient in number of patients to yield a statistically significant result (Goldschmidt 1986; Mullen and Ramirez 1987). Meta-analyses have been used, for example, to obtain estimates of the effectiveness of coronary artery bypass surgery (Wortman and Yeaton 1983) and long-term anti-arrhythmic therapy after myocardial infarction (Hine et al. 1989).

Cross-sectional studies

Nonexperiments, chiefly cross-sectional studies of populations, characterize the bulk of the literature on the effectiveness of medical care. These studies are observational, use existing registries or data bases such as the Medicare data base, apply statistical adjustments for case-mix differences, and often lack comparison groups. They are, however, more feasible, and draw upon large volumes of data reflecting actual experience. The main problem is that these data bases may have significant biases which may limit the generalizability of study results to the entire population. Most of the studies of the effectiveness of medical care, and thus much of the evidence about effectiveness to be presented and reviewed in the next section of this chapter, derive from these cross-sectional designs.

Decision analysis

Decision analyses synthesize information about effectiveness to determine the value of one approach versus another for policy analysis and ultimately for clinical decisions. A decision analysis requires information on the actual treatment of patients with disease, the outcomes, and how patients value those outcomes. Information from large data bases is used to estimate the probabilities of different outcomes from therapy for patients. Patient surveys provide information on patients' symptoms as well as their preferences for different outcomes. The advantage of a decision analysis is that it synthesizes a large amount of information relevant to effectiveness. The disadvantage is that necessary data on patient values, or preferences, are often not available. An example of a decision analysis using national-level Medicare data concerning the most effective treatment for benign prostatic hypertrophy is presented in the next section (Wennberg et al. 1988).

Data sources

Where clinical trials and true experiments are not possible, effectiveness research relies on a variety of data sources for the cross-sectional type studies mentioned earlier. These include population and provider surveys as well as birth, death, and disease registries supported by the government; and medical records data accessed through both claims data and hospital discharge data sources, many of them used for quality assurance procedures (refer again to left-hand column of Table 2.4). Several of these sources were discussed earlier in the context of population-based health status measures.

Information is also gathered by the National Health Interview Survey on respondents' use of medical care. Provider surveys, such as the National Ambulatory Medical Care Survey and the National Long-Term Care Survey, provide aggregate information on patients and their use of facilities.

Diseases are also recorded in national registries, some maintained by the government and some by private sources. An example of the former is the National Cancer Institute's Surveillance Epidemiology and End Results (SEER) system.

The majority of effectiveness research studies, however, rely on medical records and related sources such as claims data collected for billing purposes and hospital discharge abstract data collected principally for quality assurance purposes. The largest single source of claims data is the HCFA Medicare data base, of which the Medicare Provider Analysis and Review (MEDPAR) file is the most used. In addition, HCFA, through state-level peer review organizations, gathers medical record–level information about the quality of care, and is now attempting to gather this information more systematically through its planned Uniform Clinical Data Set (Krakauer and Bailey 1991). Private insurers, such as Blue Cross and Blue Shield, also maintain large claims data bases, but their usefulness is limited by the fact that there are over 1,500 private insurers in this country. In addition, these sources gather information only on patients who have health insurance.

Hospital discharge data, which are collected voluntarily for quality assurance purposes, provide another rich source of data for effectiveness research. Since the early 1950s, hospitals have voluntarily participated in the Professional Activities Study (PAS) of the Commission on Professional and Hospital Activities (CPHA). Hospitals participating in this service, for which they pay, provide discharge abstract information to CPHA, which assembles the data, summarizes it, and provides reports to participating hospitals. The data are also compiled in a central data base from which normative data are provided to member hospitals to allow them to evaluate their performance relative to other similar hospitals.

Pennsylvania, Colorado, and Iowa have mandated that all insurers and hospitals contribute to state-level data bases on hospital-level activities (Iezzoni, Schwartz, and Restuccia 1991). In addition, these states are requiring hospitals to adopt a uniform risk-adjustment method, the MedisGroups system, to accompany their data. This provides another potential source for effectiveness research.

Finally, JCAHO is also creating a national hospital data base derived from its new clinical indicators. For a common set of clinical indicators, all hospitals will provide JCAHO with information on their experience. These data will be used for accreditation decisions. The compiled data will be reported to each hospital to allow it to measure their performance against others and to seek improvements in their quality where appropriate (O'Leary 1987).

While there would appear to be great potential here, a review of claims and discharge data reveals that they have both strengths and weaknesses. The strengths include the possible linking of large data bases, the large numbers of patients included, the reliability of the factual information, and the usefulness for documenting variations in practices as well as a range of outcomes. The weaknesses are that important research variables may be missing, there is usually little information for risk adjustment, and generally postdischarge data are missing. In addition, access to the data bases is severely limited (Blumberg 1991; Jencks 1990).

In this chapter, effectiveness has been defined in terms of two complementary views, a population perspective and a clinical perspective. The population view asks what contributions medical care makes to the health of the population. The clinical view, by contrast, asks how medical care improves the health of patients who enter the system for care. The key methods of effectiveness research, which help provide answers to these questions have been described, and discussed in terms of their strengths and weaknesses. The next chapter illustrates how several of these methods—health status and severity-of-illness measurement, meta-analysis, and decision analysis—can be usefully applied in answering the basic effectiveness questions.

References

Bergner, M., R. Bobbitt, W. Carter, and B. Gilson. 1981. "The Sickness Impact Profile: Development and Final Revision of a Health Status Measure." *Medical Care* 19: 787–805.

Berkman, L., and L. Breslow. 1983. *Health and Ways of Living: The Alameda County Study.* New York: Oxford University Press.

Beta-Blocker Heart Attack Study Group. 1982. "A Randomized Trial of Propranolol in Patients with Acute Myocardial Infarction. I. Mortality Results." *Journal of the American Medical Association* 247: 1707–14.

Block, P., I. Ockene, R. Goldberg, J. Butterly, E. Block, C. Degon, A. Beiser, and T. Colton. 1988. "A Prospective Randomized Trial of Outpatient versus Inpatient Cardiac Catheterization." *New England Journal of Medicine* 319: 1251–55.

Blumberg, M. 1991. "Potentials and Limitations of Database Research Illustrated by the QMMP AMI Medicare Mortality Study." *Statistics in Medicine* 10: 637–46.

Brewster, A., B. Karlin, L. Hyde, C. Jacobs, R. Bradbury, and Y. Chae. 1985. "MEDISGRPS: A Clinically Based Approach to Classifying Hospital Patients at Admission." *Inquiry* 22: 377–87.

Brook, R. 1974. *Quality of Care Assessment: A Comparison of Five Methods of Peer Review.* DHEW-HRA-74-3100. Washington, DC: U.S. Government Printing Office.

Brook, R., and K. Lohr. 1985. "Efficacy, Effectiveness, Variations, and Quality: Boundary-Crossing Research." *Medical Care* 23 (supp.): 710–22.

Brook, R., J. Ware, W. Rogers, E. Keeler, A. Davies, C. Donald, G. Goldberg, K. Lohr, P. Masthay, and J. Newhouse. 1983. "Does Free Care Improve Adults' Health? Results from a Randomized Controlled Trial." *New England Journal of Medicine* 309: 1426–34, 1453.

Canner, P., K. Berge, N. Wenger, J. Stamler, L. Friedman, R. Prineas, and W. Friedewald. 1986. "Fifteen Year Mortality in Coronary Drug Project Patients: Long-term Benefit with Niacin." *Journal of the American College of Cardiology* 8: 1245–55.

Carlson, R. 1975. *The End of Medicine.* New York: John Wiley & Sons.

Cochrane, A. 1971. *Effectiveness and Efficiency.* London: Nuffield Provincial Hospitals Trust.

Donabedian, A. 1966. "Evaluating the Quality of Medical Care." *Milbank Memorial Fund Quarterly* 44 (Part 2): 166–206.

———. 1973. *Aspects of Medical Care Administration: Specifying Requirements for Health Care.* Cambridge, MA: Harvard University Press.

———. 1980. *Explorations in Quality Assessment and Monitoring. Volume I, The Definition of Quality and Approaches to Its Assessment.* Ann Arbor: Health Administration Press.

———. 1982. *Explorations in Quality Assessment and Monitoring. Volume II, The Criteria and Standards of Quality.* Ann Arbor: Health Administration Press.

———. 1988. "Quality Assessment and Assurance: Unity of Purpose, Diversity of Means." *Inquiry* 25: 173–92.

Dubois, R., W. Rogers, J. Moxley, D. Draper, and R. Brook. 1987. "Hospital Inpatient Mortality: Is It a Predictor of Quality?" *New England Journal of Medicine* 317: 1674–80.

Dubos, R. 1959. *Mirage of Health.* New York: Harper & Row.

Ellwood, P. 1988. "Shattuck Lecture—Outcomes Management: A Technology of Patient Experience." *New England Journal of Medicine* 318: 1549–56.

Evans, R., and G. Stoddart. 1990. "Producing Health, Consuming Health Care." *Social Science and Medicine* 31: 1347–63.

Fuchs, V. 1974. *Who Shall Live?* New York: Basic Books.

Geehr, E. 1989. *Selecting a Proprietary Severity-of-Illness System.* Tampa, FL: American College of Physician Executives.

Goldschmidt, P. 1986. "Information Synthesis: A Practical Guide." *Health Services Research* 21: 215–37.

Hansluwka, H. 1985. "Measuring the Health of Populations: Indicators and Interpretations." *Social Science and Medicine* 20: 1207–24.

HDFP. 1979. "Five-year Findings of the Hypertension Detection and Follow-up Program. I. Reduction in Mortality of Persons with High Blood Pressure, Including Mild Hypertension." *Journal of the American Medical Association* 242: 2562–71.

Health Care Financing Administration. 1986. *Medicare Hospital Mortality Information 1984.* Washington, DC: U.S. Government Printing Office.

———. 1987. *Medicare Hospital Mortality Information 1986.* Washington, DC: U.S. Government Printing Office.

Hine, L., N. Laird, P. Hewitt, and T.C. Chalmers. 1989. "Meta-analysis of Empirical Long-term Antiarrhythmic Therapy after Myocardial Infarction." *Journal of the American Medical Association* 262: 3037–40.

Horn, S., and R. Horn. 1986. "The Computerized Severity Index: A New Tool for Case-Mix Management." *Journal of Medical Systems* 10: 73–78.

Hornbrook, M. 1982. "Hospital Case Mix: Its Definition, Measurement, and Use. Part I. The Conceptual Framework. Part II. Review of Alternative Measures." *Medical Care Review* 39: 1–43, 73–123.

Iezzoni, L. 1990. "Severity of Illness Measures—Comments and Caveats." *Medical Care* 28: 757–61.

Iezzoni, L., A. Ash, G. Coffman, and M. Moskowitz. 1991. "Admission and Mid-stay MedisGroups Scores as Predictors of Death within 30 Days of Hospital Admission." *American Journal of Public Health* 81: 74–78.

Iezzoni, L., M. Schwartz, and J. Restuccia. 1991. "The Role of Severity Information in Health Policy Debates: A Survey of State and Regional Concerns." *Inquiry* 28: 117–28.

Illich, I. 1975. *Medical Nemesis.* London: M Boyars.

Jencks, S. 1990. "Issues in the Use of Large Databases for Effectiveness Research." In *Effectiveness and Outcomes in Health Care,* edited by K. A. Heithoff and K. Lohr, 94–104. Washington, DC: National Academy Press.

Kaplan, R., and J. Bush. 1982. "Health-Related Quality of Life Measurement for Evaluation Research and Policy Analysis." *Health Psychology* 1: 61–80.

Knaus, W., E. Draper, and D. Wagner. 1985. "APACHE II: A Severity of Disease Classification System." *Critical Care Medicine* 13: 818–29.

Knowles, J. 1977. "Doing Better and Feeling Worse: Health in the United States." *Daedalus* 106 (1): 1–278.

Krakauer, H., and C. Bailey. 1991. "Epidemiologic Oversight of the Medical Care Provided to Medicare Beneficiaries." *Statistics in Medicine* 10: 521–40.

Luft, H., J. Bunker, and A. Enthoven. 1979. "Should Operations be Regionalized? The Empirical Relation between Surgical Volume and Mortality." *New England Journal of Medicine* 301: 1364–69.

Martini, C., G. J. B. Allan, J. Davison, and E. M. Backett. 1977. "Health Indexes Sensitive to Medical Care Variation." *International Journal of Health Services* 7: 293–309.

McDowell, I., and C. Newell. 1987. *Measuring Health: A Guide to Rating Scales and Questionnaires.* New York: Oxford University Press.

McKeown, T. 1976. *The Role of Medicine: Dream, Mirage, or Nemesis?* London: Nuffield Provincial Hospitals Trust.

McKinlay, J., and S. McKinlay. 1977. "The Questionable Contribution of Medical Measures to the Decline of Mortality in the United States in the Twentieth Century." *Milbank Memorial Fund Quarterly* 55: 405–28.

Meenan, R., P. Gertman, and J. Mason. 1980. "Measuring Health Status in Arthritis: The Arthritis Impact Measurement Scales." *Arthritis and Rheumatism* 23: 146–52.

Milio, N. 1983. *Primary Care and the Public's Health.* Lexington, MA: Lexington Books.

Mor, V., M. Stalker, R. Gralla, et al. 1988. "Day Hospital as an Alternative to Inpatient Care for Cancer Patients: A Random Assignment Trial." *Journal of Clinical Epidemiology* 41: 771–85.

Moriyama, I., and M. Gover. 1948. "Statistical Studies of Heart Diseases. I. Heart Diseases and Allied Causes of Death in Relation to Age Changes in the Population." *Public Health Reports* 63: 537–45.

Mullen, P., and G. Ramirez. 1987. "Information Synthesis and Meta-analysis." In *Advances in Health Education and Promotion*, edited by W. Ward, M. Becker, P. Mullen, and S. Simonds, 201–39. Greenwich, CN: JAI Press.

National Center for Health Statistics. 1992. *Health, United States, 1991.* DHHS Pub. No. PHS 92-1232. Washington, DC: U.S. Government Printing Office.

O'Leary, D. 1987. "The Joint Commission Looks to the Future." *Journal of the American Medical Association* 258: 951–52.

Patrick, D. L., and R. A. Deyo. 1989. "Generic and Disease-Specific Measures in Assessing Health Status and Quality of Life." *Medical Care* 27 (supp.): S217–32.

Relman, A. 1988. "Assessment and Accountability: The Third Revolution in Medical Care." *New England Journal of Medicine* 319: 1220–22.

Sackett, D. L. 1980. "Evaluation of Health Services." In *Maxcy-Rosenau Public Health and Preventive Medicine*, edited by J. Last. Norwalk, CN: Appleton-Century-Crofts.

Stewart, A., R. Hays, and J. Ware. 1988. "The MOS Short-Form General Health

Survey: Reliability and Validity in a Patient Population." *Medical Care* 26: 724–35.

Thomas, J., and M. Ashcraft. 1991. "Measuring Severity of Illness: Six Severity Systems and Their Ability to Explain Cost Variations." *Inquiry* 28 (1): 39–55.

VA Cooperative Study Group. 1970. "Effects of Treatment on Morbidity in Hypertension. II. Results in Patients with Diastolic Blood Pressure Averaging 90 through 114 mm Hg." *Journal of the American Medical Association* 213: 1143–52.

Wennberg, J. 1984. "Dealing with Medical Practice Variations: A Proposal for Action." *Health Affairs* 3 (2): 6–32.

———. 1990. "Small Area Analysis and the Medical Care Outcome Problem." In *Research Methodology: Strengthening Causal Interpretations of Nonexperimental Data*, edited by L. Sechrest, B. Starfield, and J. Bunker. Rockville, MD: Agency for Health Care Policy and Research.

Wennberg, J., and A. Gittelsohn. 1973. "Small Area Variations in Health Care Delivery." *Science* 182: 1102–8.

Wennberg, J., A. Mulley, D. Hanley, R. Timothy, F. Fowler, N. Roos, M. Barry, K. McPherson, E. R. Greenber, D. Soule, T. Bubolz, E. Fisher, and D. Malenka. 1988. "An Assessment of Prostatectomy for Benign Urinary Tract Obstruction: Geographic Variations and the Evaluation of Medical Care Outcomes." *Journal of the American Medical Association* 259: 3027–30.

Williamson, J. 1978. *Assessing and Improving Health Care Outcomes: The Health Accounting Approach to Quality Assurance*. Cambridge, MA: Ballinger Publishing Company.

Williamson, J., M. Alexander, and G. Miller. 1968. "Priorities in Patient-Care Research and Continuing Medical Education." *Journal of the American Medical Association* 204: 93–98.

Williamson, J., D. Moore, and P. Sanazaro. 1991. "Moving from 'Small qa' to "LARGE QA": An Outcomes Framework for Improving Quality Management." *Evaluation and the Health Professions* 14 (2): 138–60.

Woolsey, T., and I. Moriyama. 1948. "Statistical Studies of Heart Diseases II. Important Factors in Heart Disease Mortality Trends." *Public Health Reports* 63: 1247–73.

Wortman, P., and W. Yeaton. 1983. "Synthesis of Results in Controlled Trials of Coronary Artery Bypass Graft Surgery." *Evaluation Studies, Review Annual* 8: 536–51.

Effectiveness: Evidence and an Application

This chapter reviews the evidence that answers the two primary research questions concerning effectiveness: what are the contributions of medical care to the health of the population; and can the clinical effectiveness of medical care be improved? Following this review, a policy-related application of effectiveness research, i.e., outcomes assessment, will be described and explored.

Evidence Relating to the Effectiveness of Medical Care

The effectiveness questions concern the contributions of medical care to health. In light of the ideas represented in Table 2.1, this general question can be broken down into several more specific questions concerning the relationships between the structures and processes of medical care and the outcomes of medical care. The questions concerning the relationships between *structure and outcomes* are these:

— Is there evidence that the *efficacy of medical care interventions* is related to outcomes?

— Is there evidence that the *quantity of medical care resources* explains variations in outcomes?

— Is there evidence that improved *distribution of and access to* medical care improves health status outcomes for populations?

The questions concerning the relationships between *processes and outcomes* are these:

— Is there evidence that increased *use of medical care* contributes to improved outcomes?

— Is there evidence that the *quantity of medical care procedures* done relates to variations in outcomes?

— Is there evidence that the *quality of the medical care* makes a difference in the results of the care?

Selected evidence related to each of these questions will be presented separately for the population and the clinical perspectives. It is not the intent of this chapter to review comprehensively all of the evidence bearing on these questions. Rather, selected examples illustrate the types of evidence and the general weight of the evidence.

Improving the health of the population

Efficacy and population outcomes

While the randomized clinical trial is the principal method for determining the efficacy of medical care interventions, the following example illustrates the creative use of a cross-sectional study design, in this case, observations over time, to assess the effectiveness of medical care given efficacious therapies for the conditions under consideration.

As mentioned earlier, between the early and late 1900s in this country there was a dramatic shift in mortality from deaths due to acute infectious diseases to deaths due to chronic disease such as heart disease, cancer, and strokes. This dramatic shift was assumed to be due to the introduction of antibiotics to cure the acute infectious diseases and vaccines to prevent their occurrence. Using mortality data over this time period, available from U.S. Vital Statistics sources, McKinlay and McKinlay (1977) set out to test this hypothesis. They examined the data for ten common infectious diseases: tuberculosis, scarlet fever, influenza, pneumonia, diphtheria, whooping cough, measles, smallpox, typhoid fever, and poliomyelitis. They demonstrated that for every condition they examined, except for smallpox, most of the decline in mortality from the disease had occurred before the introduction of the antibiotic or the vaccine specific for that disease. For the ten diseases they examined, the average net reduction in mortality after the introduction of the disease-specific intervention was 25 percent, although the range was from 0.29 percent for typhoid fever to 100 percent for smallpox. Even for poliomyelitis, the decline following the 1955 introduction of the Salk and Sabin vaccines was a modest 25 percent. In other words, specific medical interventions appear to have made only small contributions to the decline in mortality from the acute infectious diseases in this country.

This study and others similar to it (Charlton and Velez 1986) reveal only marginal benefits from efficacious medical care.

Quantity and population outcomes

Besides efficacy, the relationship between the quantity of resources and outcomes has been explored in studies with nonexperimental designs using cross-sectional observational data. Cochrane, St. Leger, and Moore (1978), using various mortality rates from 18 developed nations as the outcomes, and resource-to-population rates as the structural variables, found no consistent relationship of mortality to the levels of medical care resources. In fact, mortality rates were most sensitive to the GNP-per-person and physician-to-population rates, but in opposite directions. Higher GNPs were associated with lower mortality rates, but the higher the number of physicians per population, the higher the mortality rate. This paradoxical effect—more physicians are related to greater death rates—has since been explored, but not explained. The expected effect was found for nurses, however, with greater nurse-to-population ratios being associated with lower mortality rates.

Newhouse and Friedlander (1979) found disease-prevalence rates from the U.S. Health and Nutrition Examination Survey were unrelated to the levels of medical care resources across census regions. They examined the prevalence of hypertension, varicose veins, high cholesterol levels, abnormal electrocardiograms, and abnormal x-rays, in relation to the distribution of primary care physicians, all physicians, dentists, and hospital beds per population. The only statistically significant association they found was for all physicians and hypertension, but it, too, was in the opposite direction of what was predicted, i.e., more physicians were associated with a greater prevalence of hypertension. Each of these studies confirms the suggestion that medical care makes only a modest contribution to the health of the population, whether the outcome measure is mortality or disease prevalence and whether the comparison is across countries or within a single country.

Distribution and population outcomes

It has been suggested that it is not merely the quantity of medical care resources, but their distribution, that is important to the health of the population. Using city health department data in an analytic study design, Gordis (1973) determined the effect of the presence of comprehensive community health centers on the incidence of rheumatic fever in Baltimore. He found a lower incidence of rheumatic fever among children in the geographic areas of the city that had comprehensive community health centers, the assumption being that these children had better access to definitive treatment with penicillin.

An observational study done using longitudinal data from England investigated the effect of improving the distribution of health care resources on population mortality rates (Hollingsworth 1981). The author used data from before and after the introduction of the National Health Service to determine the effect of changing the distribution of medical care resources on population mortality rates by social class. He found that, despite the achievement of equity in distribution of health care resources by geographic health region, increased use of services by lower social class patients, and improvements in mortality rates, differences in health status between those at opposite ends of the socioeconomic scale persisted after nearly 40 years of experience in the British National Health Service. For example, the data show that, while overall neonatal mortality rates declined over 50 percent during this period of time, the difference in neonatal mortality by social class increased by 25 percent for the lowest social class relative to the highest by 1972.

Process and population outcomes

Evidence relating to process and outcomes includes studies examining the relationships between the process variables of utilization, quantity of procedures, and quality of care, and various outcome variables.

The RAND Health Insurance Experiment (Brook et al. 1983) provides the best example of the examination of the effects of varying utilization rates upon health outcomes. This study was designed as a prospective experiment with families from six different communities across the United States randomly allocated to different payment groups. The study was undertaken to determine what influence various levels of copayment in a national health insurance scheme might have, primarily on utilization and secondarily on health status. The utilization examined in this study included outpatient and inpatient care for adults and children. The clinical outcomes assessed were blood pressure and vision for adults; anemia, hay fever, hearing, fluid in the middle ear, and vision for children. Utilization was 33 percent greater for adults and 22 percent greater for children in the free care plan than in the 95 percent copay plan (Valdez et al. 1985). These utilization differences accompanied only slight differences in blood pressure and vision correction in the adults and no differences in clinical outcomes in the children. One conclusion is that medical care makes only a modest contribution to the health of people based on selected clinical measures. For the lower income families in this study, the results were more dramatic; even modest levels of coinsurance adversely affected their health (Brook 1991).

A cross-sectional study conducted in Boston and New Haven reached a similar conclusion of marginal benefits for greater investment of resources (Wennberg et al. 1989). Using Medicare data, Wennberg and his colleagues showed that, despite utilization and costs being twice as high for hospitals in Boston, the outcomes in terms of Medicare beneficiary mortality rates did not differ. Initial severity of illness and other demographics did not appear to explain the differences in utilization.

Summary

Overall there is evidence that medical care, whether measured by its structural or process aspects, and whether measured at the individual, institutional, system, or national level, contributes only modestly to the health of the population. One problem with this conclusion is that the preponderance of the evidence is based on observational data and cross-sectional designs. These are weaker study designs in that they cannot make clear the direction of effects, and their potential causes. The one exception is the RAND study, which used an experimental design with an intervention *followed* by an assessment of effects, and random allocation of subjects. The former design characteristic clarifies the direction of the effects, while the latter controls for the other possible causes.

Furthermore, most of these studies have used mortality as their outcome, and mortality has repeatedly been shown to be more highly correlated with environmental and sociodemographic variables than with medical care (Martini et al. 1977). This makes mortality not only less sensitive to medical care variation, but subject to confounding by other factors. In addition, appropriate risk adjustments are usually not possible (the necessary data are not available in mortality data sets) in making comparisons on mortality between groups. This omission makes it difficult to distinguish outcomes of medical care from the initial condition of patients.

The Medical Outcomes Study was undertaken to address these issues and to define better the contribution of medical care to patient outcomes (Tarlov et al. 1989). The Medical Outcomes Study uses the structure-process-outcome conceptual framework and combines both cross-sectional and longitudinal designs in the same study. The study examines systems of care, styles of practice, specialty issues, and outcomes for the poor and elderly in the context of this framework. It examines system, provider, and patient characteristics as the structural variables; technical and interpersonal style as the process variables; and clinical end points, functional status, general well-being, and satisfaction with care as the outcomes. A longitudinal part of the study is designed to follow diabetes, hypertension, coronary heart disease, and depression patients in Boston, Chicago, and Los Angeles to relate the structural and process variables to the full range of outcomes specified above.

Published results demonstrate differences in functional health status measures among patients with different chronic medical conditions (Stewart et al. 1989). These results assure the validity of the health status measures being used and confirm the need to use more than just clinical outcomes to assess the effectiveness of medical care. The study has the potential to provide more definitive evidence pertaining to the effects of provider and system characteristics on the outcomes of care.

Improving the effectiveness of medical care

The important health policy and health services research question regarding effectiveness at the present time is, can the effectiveness of medical care be improved? The investigation of this question begins with randomized clinical trials to determine the efficacy of procedures and, hence, the standard against which actual medical practice can be compared. To the degree that the results in actual clinical practice, i.e, effectiveness, fall short of the levels determined by efficacy studies, it is assumed there is room for improvement. Hypertension provides one example of the use of this approach.

Efficacy and clinical outcomes

A randomized clinical trial (RCT) of male veterans with hypertension was carried out in the 1960s. Specific drug therapy was contrasted with the effectiveness of placebo treatment in men with hypertension. The results in the moderate hypertensive group, using mortality and morbidity as the outcome measures, were conclusive at the end of the trial. Systematic drug treatment for hypertension was effective in reducing mortality and morbidity from the disease (VA Cooperative Study Group 1970). This study and its positive results represent an example of a prototype study of a medical intervention, whether medication or procedural, and the determination of its efficacy.

The Hypertension Detection and Follow-up Program (HDFP) was undertaken to determine whether the findings of the VA study applied to the general population and to patients with mild hypertension (HDFP 1979). It can also be interpreted as a study designed to determine the magnitude of the gap between efficacy and effectiveness. Five-year total mortality rates were compared between those subjects allocated to the ideal protocol derived from the VA study and those subjects assigned to usual, or referred, care. The study demonstrated a significant reduction in five-year total mortality for the subjects under the ideal protocol, clearly demonstrating that better-quality medical care produces better outcomes and that the effectiveness of medical care for the treatment of hypertension might be improved.

More recent work on hypertension, however, has confirmed the limits of the improvements that can be expected (Bonita and Beaglehole 1989). Epidemiological studies have shown that the clinical trials of efficacy underestimated the benefits of hypertension treatment by as much as 10 percent, but they have also demonstrated that as much as 75 percent of the decline in adverse hypertension outcomes is unrelated to specific treatments.

Quantity and clinical outcomes

Once the efficacy of procedures has been established, the effects of greater quantities of procedures on outcomes can also be examined. An example of such a study is one that examined the relationship between the number of surgical procedures done in hospitals and each hospital's mortality experience for those operations. Using adjusted case fatality rates by hospital as the outcome, and frequency of the surgical procedure as the process variable, the researchers (Luft, Bunker, and Enthoven 1979) showed that greater frequency of procedures is associated with better outcomes, i.e., lower mortality rates. For example, for coronary bypass surgery, they showed that hospitals that do more than 200 procedures per year had lower mortality rates. The same threshold level of 200 held for vascular and prostate surgery. For other surgeries, the threshold volume level was much lower: 50 for bowel surgery and total hip replacement, and 10 for gallbladder surgery. A later review of the several studies of this type confirmed the basic findings (Office of Technology Assessment 1988). The implication of such studies is that the effectiveness of medical care, for surgical procedures, can be improved. One suggestion of these authors and others is to regionalize surgery for the procedures requiring a high volume to maximize effectiveness. There is, however, a continuing debate over whether these differences are truly the result of differences in medical care quality, or whether they result from differences in referral patterns. It is conceivable that the institutions with better mortality results began with patients in less serious condition.

Quality and clinical outcomes

A similar question has been investigated with regard to the variation in hospital mortality rates for various medical conditions. Using a cross-sectional design and a hospital data base, investigators (Dubois et al. 1987) examined the relationship between hospital mortality rates for three specific conditions—heart attack, pneumonia, and stroke—and two different measures of quality of care. They found that 64 percent of the variation in outcomes was explained by the severity of illness of patients upon admission to these hospitals, but that there was an association between poorer quality and mortality for one quality assessment method (based on a subjective judgment of preventability of death). A subsequent study (Park et al. 1990) confirmed the finding of a modest inverse association between the quality of medical care given and the subsequent death of individual patients.

The variations evidence

Other evidence relating to evaluations of the clinical effectiveness of medical care, first presented by Wennberg and Gittelsohn (1973) and confirmed many times over in different locations and with different procedures and methods, indicates substantial variation in patterns of clinical practice. Population-based rates of surgical procedures, such as tonsillectomy and adenoidectomy, appendectomy, hysterectomy, and herniorrhaphy vary by as much as 5- and 6-fold from one geographic area to another (Wennberg 1984). The rates for diagnostic procedures vary among Medicare recipients across the country as much as 10- to 30-fold (Chassin, Brook, and Park 1986). Rates of hospital utilization and expenditures for Medicare patients show a 2-fold variation between the seemingly comparable hospital service areas of Boston and New Haven (Wennberg et al. 1989).

While the evidence of variation is abundant, the interpretation of these differences has resisted clarification. It has been argued that the differences may be a statistical artifact of the small areas analyzed, with the estimates being unstable and not comparable because of population differences (Wennberg 1990b). While age adjustment of the variations data has been used to control for probable population differences in health status, Blumberg holds that age is not a good proxy for health status (Blumberg 1987). Wennberg and his colleagues have responded to these and other challenges to the variations evidence with improved analyses and more appropriate statistical adjustments (Wennberg 1987; Wennberg 1990b). The result is that, while the magnitude of the variations is reduced, the differences cannot be explained away. There are real variations, and they suggest room for improving the effectiveness of medical care.

Summary

Quality of care and mortality studies suggest, as do the HDFP and surgical volume studies, that there is room for improving the effectiveness of medical care. The HDFP confirmed that the gap between efficacy and effectiveness can have significant consequences in mortality for patients. The surgical volume studies would appear to corroborate the benefits of better medical care, and several studies confirm the importance of better quality for enhanced, but modest improvements in, outcomes. The epidemiologic studies of hypertension and the studies of hospital mortality and quality, however, emphasize the modest improvements resulting directly from better or improved medical care.

In essence, then, we have a substantial body of evidence that suggests that medical care does indeed make a modest contribution to the health of the population. We have some evidence that the effectiveness of medical care can be improved, and we have evidence of wide variation in medical practice that is as yet unexplained. The question of concern is whether these variations are associated with differences in outcomes. If certain procedures or interventions are clearly of benefit, they should be adopted and noneffective ones dropped. Most medical interventions carry some risk, and if the risk associated with a procedure does not justify the benefits, then it should be abandoned.

An Application: Outcomes Assessment

These findings raise additional questions about what can be done to improve effectiveness, but the answers proposed depend upon the level of focus. At the population level, with medical care viewed as only one of the inputs to the health of the population, then we can ask whether investment in medical care is the best way to improve the health of the population. By contrast, if we view the structures and processes of medical care as the important foci for improving the health of the population and thus emphasize the medical care system level, we might ask if the effectiveness of medical care can be improved through manipulation of system-level variables. Finally, if we direct our attention to the clinical level, then we might ask what can be done to influence individual provider and patient behaviors.

These levels of focus and their implications lead to quite different proposals in terms of deciding what is the problem to be addressed and what are the appropriate solutions. For example, if the population level is the focus, the proposals favor reducing investments in medical care and focusing on changing harmful lifestyles through public policy (Breslow 1972; Evans and Stoddart 1990; Fuchs 1974; Milio 1983). Milio's arguments in favor of "using public policy tools for health promotion, as illustrated with farm-food-cigarette policies" (Milio 1983, 111) reflect this approach. Specifically, she proposes using farm subsidies to alter what foods are produced, for example more healthy ones, and to replace tobacco with other crops. Such an approach might be viewed as the health promotion–disease prevention initiative that has clamored for attention for a couple of decades beginning in the 1960s with the ascending mortality rates from chronic disease and their seeming resistance to decline. Public opinion in response to these problems was that investments in medical care were not producing improvements in health, so efforts should be directed toward promoting healthier lifestyles.

The earlier advocates of health promotion (Breslow 1972; Fuchs 1974; Knowles 1977; Lalonde 1975; Surgeon General 1979) saw some of their ideas implemented and some policies changed, but, overall, medicine was not to be displaced as the means of solving this society's health problems. Furthermore, the rapid and significant decline in mortality rates that began in the late 1960s was interpreted in many quarters as a medical care success. Evans and Stoddart (1990) also argue that medicine co-opted much of this movement through individual risk factor management, and that is why it has been largely ineffective. They further contend that social problems cause poor health, that social problems cannot be addressed by medical care, and that policymakers have been resistant to choosing any other approach.

If, however, medical care is assumed to be the way to improve the health of the population, i.e., its effectiveness for this purpose is not questioned, and if the focus is on the system level, then proposals for improving medical care target system-level variables. For example, Wennberg, reflecting an idea that had an earlier incarnation in the form of comprehensive health planning, argues that we should not try to micromanage the practice of medicine by physicians, i.e., by specifying practice guidelines, but that instead we should limit the resources put into medical care in the form of hospital beds and expensive technology (Wennberg 1990b). By limiting capacity, he claims, we can effectively address both the tendency for demand to expand to meet supply and the temptation of physicians to try anything to help their patients, even when patients do not demand it.

When, however, neither the population nor the system focus holds policymakers' attention, and yet they are concerned with both the effectiveness and costs of medical care, the solutions that emerge center on the clinical practice of physicians themselves. The proposals generated range from the more modest ones of national quality improvement initiatives funded by a portion of medical care insurance to those implicit in the legislation that funded the Agency for Health Care Policy and Research, i.e., clinical practice guidelines.

The approach to improving quality through professional standards review organizations that originated in the 1970s is now in the midst of a reformulation. For example, the proposals of the National Leadership

Commission on Health Care (1989) embody a quality-focused effort. The commission's initiative proposed to expand the national information base about quality, promote the development of practice guidelines, and foster the dissemination of these guidelines through information and incentives, all of this being funded by a surtax on health insurance premiums paid by both employees and their employers.

The legislation setting up the AHCPR proposed mechanisms for the development and dissemination of practice guidelines, i.e., specifications of what procedures should and should not be used by all physicians in the treatment of patients with specific conditions. In the most general sense, this latter approach is the embodiment of what has become known as outcomes assessment and management (Ellwood 1988; Wennberg 1990a, 1990b), where assessment refers to effectiveness research focused on outcomes, and management implies the development, dissemination, and application of practice guidelines.

Outcomes assessment and management

Theory and methods

Of the various alternatives and proposals, outcomes assessment and management seems to have gained the spotlight and the lion's share of funding for the present. It appears sufficiently strong for Relman (1988) to herald it as ushering in the Era of Accountability. Wennberg's leadership in developing the science has been influential in bringing outcomes assessment and management to the public policy level.

In a sense, the work that Wennberg and his colleague Gittelsohn began (Wennberg and Gittelsohn 1973) culminated in the creation of the Agency for Health Care Policy and Research with its agenda devoted to outcomes assessment and management. This agency made the effectiveness of medical care a primary public policy goal. For that reason, the remainder of this chapter explores the assumptions, the implementation, and examples of this new approach which has now been embodied in a $50-million-a-year enterprise (Raskin and Maklan 1991).

Two principal assumptions behind this assessment and management effort are articulated in an article written by two AHCPR staff members (Raskin and Maklan 1991, 164): "(1) Variations in clinical practice are associated with differences in patient outcomes and resource use, [and] (2) Inappropriate practice patterns can be changed if relevant scientific evidence is effectively disseminated to health care providers and patients." Furthermore, the underlying assumption for all of this effort is that medical care does indeed contribute substantially to improving the health of the population.

The first assumption is certainly true for differences in resource use, but it has yet to be proven for differences in patient outcomes. Several examples presented in the evidence section of this chapter would question the validity of this part of the assumption. The work of Dubois et al. (1987) and Park et al. (1990) found little if any relationship between variations in quality and differences in outcomes. Wennberg's work with benign prostatic hypertrophy found little difference in outcomes despite the major contrast involved in "watchful waiting versus immediate surgery" (Barry et al. 1988). His work comparing Boston and New Haven (Wennberg et al. 1989) found no real differences in outcomes despite twofold variations in resource use.

The second assumption, regarding the possibility for changing practice patterns through disseminating scientific evidence on probable treatment outcomes, will be discussed later in this section, but suffice it to say now that it is of questionable validity also.

Nonetheless, these assumptions and the work of Wennberg (Wennberg et al. 1988) have provided the basis for the AHCPR's Patient Outcome Research Team (PORT) projects, the agency's showpiece for implementing outcomes assessment and management. Each PORT is designed to apply the outcomes assessment processes to an identifiable medical condition: (1) evaluation of published evidence and current opinion to understand major controversies and identify hypotheses for further study; (2) use of large claims data bases to determine probability estimates of various outcomes; (3) prospective outcomes study through interviews with patients and their providers to assess patients' symptoms and functional status; and (4) decision analysis to provide a rational synthesis of the information for policy purposes.

The steps of outcomes assessment draw upon the key methods of effectiveness research described in the earlier section of this chapter. Published evidence is evaluated using the tools of information synthesis and meta-analysis, while prospective studies of patients' outcomes incorporate health-related quality of life measures yielding patients' valuation of outcomes. These valuations provide the utilities needed for the quality-adjusted life-years in the decision analysis. The decision analysis itself uses statistical modeling and incorporates the outcome probabilities and utilities derived from the earlier parts of the process to yield average outcomes for typical patients.

In addition to performing these outcomes assessment steps, each PORT is expected to disseminate findings about effectiveness and to use experimental designs to evaluate the effectiveness of that dissemination in changes in practice patterns as well as in improved patient outcomes. From 1989 to 1991, the AHCPR funded 12 PORT projects for five years each, to the level of about $1 million per year, to explore effectiveness relative to the following conditions: acute myocardial infarction, prostate disease, low back pain, cataracts, arthritis of the knee (total knee replacement), chronic ischemic heart disease, diabetes, gallbladder disease, pneumonia, hip fracture and osteoarthritis of the hip (total hip replacement), obstetric care (management of labor and delivery), and stroke (Raskin and Maklan 1991).

An example

The work of Wennberg on benign prostatic hypertrophy over the past decade provides an excellent example of the application of the outcomes assessment methods to studying the effectiveness of medical care as well as the dissemination and evaluation activities in developing the basis for improving that care. Wennberg, Bunker, and Barnes (1980) did the initial evaluation of published evidence as part of a review of several common conditions. They identified a controversy regarding the treatment of benign prostatic hypertrophy, between "early interventionists," who argued for early resection of the prostate, and the "conservative school," who argued for a "watchful waiting" approach to treatment. Wennberg and his colleagues spent the next decade investigating and attempting to resolve this controversy.

Wennberg et al. (1987) used large claims data bases, including U.S. Medicare data and the equivalent Canadian data base, to identify the probable outcomes and their patterns of association with structural and process variables. These studies identified hospital size and the open surgical procedure as prognostic factors for outcomes.

The prospective outcomes study was done on a sample of about 300 patients. The patients were assessed not only as to their symptoms and their severity, but, more important, for their perceptions or reactions to those symptoms (Fowler et al. 1988). What became clear was that the symptoms and their severity alone were not enough to determine how the condition would affect the quality of life of the patients. It was important also to assess specifically the impact of the symptoms on the individual patient so that the decision about surgery or watchful waiting would include the patient's preferences for what he could and could not bear, an entirely personal judgment. This result led Wennberg and his colleagues to devote considerable effort to providing the necessary information in appropriate forms to patients so that they, with their physicians, can make informed decisions about surgery.

The decision analysis part of outcomes assessment, as mentioned earlier, is undertaken to provide a rational synthesis of the information derived from the previous stages in the process. Wennberg's decision analysis incorporated the outcome probability data derived from reviews of published studies, the large data base analysis, and information about patients' quality of life judgments of their symptoms. Using the example of a 70-year-old man without other complicating health problems as the baseline, and following the modeling process for the equivalent of ten years of life for the man, the authors determined that there is a "net loss of 1.01 months of life expectancy for those who undergo immediate operation" for benign prostatic hypertrophy (Barry et al. 1988). In other words, and in contrast to the conventional wisdom that immediate surgery saves lives, for the typical man without other complications, "watchful waiting"—doing no surgery—is in the long run less likely to shorten life. On the other hand, when the quality of life is considered in the form of patients' preferences for living with certain symptoms and complications, then there is a net gain of about three quality-adjusted life-months for patients undergoing immediate surgery. In other words, when patients' valuations of symptoms are taken into account, the relief of symptoms by immediate surgery is like gaining three months of life.

Development of practice guidelines

The example of Wennberg's analysis of watchful waiting versus immediate surgery for benign prostatic hypertrophy provides an illustration of an outcomes assessment, but what the PORT process and outcomes management call for is extending this information into the development of practice guidelines, the dissemination of those guidelines, and the evaluation of the effect of that dissemination. A major part of the activities of the AHCPR is devoted to these activities. In fact, the initial legislation passed by Congress called for the agency to publish its first three sets of practice guidelines by January of 1991. It met that deadline with drafts of guidelines for urinary incontinence in adults, preventing pressure ulcers, and pain management. These underwent review and comment for a year, and were published and disseminated in final form in 1992. Also during this year, the agency began funding dissemination research projects to determine the most effective means of implementing adoption of the practice guidelines it developed.

But what exactly are practice guidelines, what are their purposes, what are their sources, how are they developed, how are they most effectively disseminated, and do they work? What the Institute of Medicine calls practice guidelines and AHCPR calls clinical guidelines have been variously referred to as practice standards (Brook 1989), clinical practice guidelines (Geehr and Salluzo 1990), practice policies (Eddy 1990a, 877), and consensus statement guidelines (Hill, Levine, and Whelton 1988). Further, the American Medical Association knows them as practice parameters, the American College of Physicians as medical necessity guidelines, and the Joint Commission on Accreditation of Healthcare Organizations as clinical indicators. Such standards are intended to guide and influence the diagnostic, procedural, and treatment decisions a physician makes toward the more appropriate and cost-effective alternatives. In fact they are, in the words of Wennberg (1990a), designed to micromanage medical care, at the level of the specific clinical encounter between a physician and an individual patient.

While practice guidelines became federal policy with the passage of PL 101-239 in 1989, they are not new, and they are not the exclusive prerogative of the federal government. Practice guidelines have been and are being developed and used by private insurers, medical specialty societies, and voluntary health care organizations as well as by governmental agencies. Federal agencies producing practice guidelines, in addition to the AHCPR, include the Centers for Disease Control, National Cancer Institute, Health Care Financing Administration, and Physician Payment Review Commission. Private payers such as Blue Cross and Blue Shield, as well as other private health insurers, have and are issuing such guidelines. Perhaps in the belief that the best defense is a good offense, the various medical specialty societies such as the American College of Physicians, the American College of Cardiology, and the American College of Obstetricians and Gynecologists have been voluntarily developing their own guidelines. Voluntary health associations such as the American Hospital Association, the American Medical Association, and the Joint Commission on Accreditation of Healthcare Organizations have adopted a similar posture. In addition, the Institute of Medicine, a quasi-governmental research organization, has produced practice guidelines in a number of areas.

Different means have been used by each of these sources, but Eddy (1990b, 1265) describes the process generically as:

— identify important health outcomes;

— analyze evidence for the effects of practice on those outcomes;

— estimate the magnitudes of the outcomes (benefits and harms);

— compare the benefits and harms;

— estimate the costs;

— compare the health outcomes with the costs; and

— compare alternative practices to determine which deserve priority.

Using such a process, guidelines have been developed and issued over the years for a number of conditions, including the 1984 Joint National

Committee Consensus Report on high blood pressure, National Consensus Development Conference on cesarean sections, and American Heart Association guidelines for prevention of bacterial endocarditis. An example of a practice guideline is shown in Table 3.1.

Evaluation of practice guidelines

Are practice guidelines effective in altering the medical practice decisions of physicians? There is only a modest body of research on practice guidelines, their effectiveness, and the determinants of their effectiveness. One operating assumption is that, once practice guidelines are developed, simply disseminating them will alter physician behaviors.

Several studies indicate that simple dissemination has almost no impact on practice decisions. One such study (Hill, Levine, and Whelton 1988) demonstrated that, while availability and awareness of the 1984 Joint National Committee Consensus Report on high blood pressure were high, actual use and medical practice were barely altered as judged by before and after questionnaires related to practice behaviors. Similar findings have been reported for other consensus statement guidelines (Brooks 1980; Gleicher 1984).

Lomas et al. (1989) found that physicians' knowledge, attitudes, and reported behavior toward a Canadian consensus statement concerning cesarean section rates and the need to decrease them were all positive, but

Table 3.1   An Example of a Practice Guideline: Follow-up Criteria for Initial Blood Pressure Measurement

Range, mm Hg	*Recommended Follow-up*
Diastolic	
<85	Recheck within 2 years
85–89	Recheck within 1 year
90–104	Confirm within 2 months
105–114	Evaluate or refer promptly to source of care within 2 weeks
>115	Evaluate or refer immediately to source of care
Systolic, when diastolic blood pressure is <90	
<140	Recheck within 2 years
140–199	Confirm within 2 months
>200	Evaluate or refer promptly to source of care within 2 weeks

Source: Joint National Committee on Detection, Evaluation, and Treatment of High Blood Pressure 1989.

the assessed rates of cesarean section before and after the distribution of the statement were up to 50 percent higher than reported and represented only a slight change from the previous upward trend.

A systematic effort in the direction of practice guidelines has been the National Institutes of Health's Consensus Development Program. Through this program the National Institutes of Health (NIH) brings together a wide range of experts to develop practice guidelines for physicians and then disseminates the recommendations though a variety of means. Kosecoff and her colleagues (1987) investigated the effectiveness of this process for 12 consensus recommendations. They found little effect from any of the recommendations, although physicians were aware of them. More important, the researchers observed that physician behaviors with regard to several of the guidelines were changing even before the consensus statements were disseminated.

Dissemination of consensus statement guidelines alone *does not* appear to alter behavior substantially. Brook (1991) has argued for the linking of practice guidelines and financial incentives. Wennberg, however, advocates feedback of information about the variations in practices and outcomes as a means of stimulating physicians themselves to engage in a process of developing guidelines. Here the effects would seem to be greater, but with the caveat that such dissemination include systematic organizational efforts at change.

Wennberg (1984) used the technique of providing the information on variations in surgical procedure rates to physicians in Vermont, Maine, and Iowa. Local leaders in medicine became engaged with the data, and led their colleagues in a re-examination of their approach to surgical treatments. Relevant literature was reviewed, and in one case, the state medical journal published the results. The efforts proved successful in reducing tonsillectomy rates in Vermont to 10 percent of their previous level. Wennberg also reports that similar efforts in the other states have proved equally effective.

Feedback of information when followed by such a systematic change process involving the relevant professional group does appear to alter physician practice patterns, evidence that prompted Wennberg (1990a, 1204) to ask and answer the following question: "Will the pressures placed on the doctor-patient relationship by managed care and practice guidelines exert sufficient influence on the supply to achieve the needed reallocation in fee-for-service markets? Everything I have learned about the peculiar relations among medical theory, the supply of resources and the practice styles of physicians in fee-for-service markets warns me that this cannot be so." Wennberg, in this statement, is arguing that micromanaging medical care through practice guidelines will not result in reducing the number of physicians, the number of hospital beds, or the quantity of expensive medical machines. He goes on to argue that only by conscious, system-level decisions to reallocate medical care dollars to appropriate resources can we achieve the necessary reduction of expenditures for medical care.

This chapter on effectiveness addresses several questions. In answer to the first question, regarding what the contributions of medical care are to the health of the population, we have a substantial body of evidence that suggests that medical care does indeed make a contribution to the health of the population but that the contribution is modest. In answer to the second question, regarding whether the clinical effectiveness of medical care can be improved, we have clear evidence of wide variation in medical practice which is unexplained and as yet not clearly related to outcomes, and we have some evidence that the effectiveness of medical care can be improved.

Of the various policy options for improving effectiveness, including health promotion (Milio 1983), health planning (Wennberg 1990b), and outcomes assessment and management (Ellwood 1988; National Leadership Commission on Health Care 1989; Wennberg 1990a, 1990b), outcomes assessment and management has become the dominant focus of federal policy on effectiveness, reflected in the research and policy agenda of the Agency for Health Care Policy and Research. But the evidence in favor of this endeavor is not entirely supportive, and two additional questions may well be posed as a result. First, how did such an activity become federal policy when the evidence to support it was not there? Second, if this outcomes assessment and management strategy is in time proven to be of limited benefit in improving medical care effectiveness, then the question still remaining will be, what can be done to improve the health of the population? At some time in the future, we may well turn our attention to a more macro-oriented approach to improving the nation's health.

References

Barry, M., A. Mulley, F. Fowler, and J. Wennberg. 1988. "Watchful Waiting vs. Immediate Transurethral Resection for Symptomatic Prostatism: The Importance of Patients' Preferences." *Journal of the American Medical Association* 259: 3010–17.

Blumberg, M. 1987. "Inter-area Variations in Age-adjusted Health Status." *Medical Care* 25: 340–53.

Bonita, R., and R. Beaglehole. 1989. "Increased Treatment of Hypertension Does Not Explain the Decline in Stroke Mortality in the United States, 1970–1980." *Hypertension* 13 (5 supp.): 169–73.

Breslow, L. 1972. "A Quantitative Approach to the World Health Organization Definition of Health: Physical, Mental and Social Well-being." *International Journal of Epidemiology* 1: 347–55.

Brook, R. 1989. "Practice Guidelines and Practicing Medicine. Are They Compatible?" *Journal of the American Medical Association* 262: 3027–30.

———. 1991. "Health, Health Insurance, and the Uninsured." *Journal of the American Medical Association* 265: 2998–3002.

Brook, R., J. Ware, W. Rogers, E. Keeler, A. Davies, C. Donald, G. Goldberg, K. Lohr, P. Masthay, and J. Newhouse. 1983. "Does Free Care Improve Adults' Health? Results from a Randomized Controlled Trial." *New England Journal of Medicine* 309: 1426–34, 1453.

Brooks, S. 1980. "Survey of Compliance with American Heart Association Guidelines for Prevention of Bacterial Endocarditis." *Journal of the American Dental Association* 101: 41–43.

Charlton, J., and R. Velez. 1986. "Some International Comparisons of Mortality Amenable to Medical Intervention." *British Medical Journal* 292: 295–301.

Chassin, M., R. Brook, and R. Park. 1986. "Variations in the Use of Medical and Surgical Services by the Medicare Population." *New England Journal of Medicine* 314: 285–90.

Cochrane, A. L., A. S. St. Leger, and F. Moore. 1978. "Health Service 'Input' and Mortality 'Output' in Developed Countries." *Journal of Epidemiology and Community Health* 32: 200–205.

Dubois, R., W. Rogers, J. Moxley, D. Draper, and R. Brook. 1987. "Hospital Inpatient Mortality: Is It a Predictor of Quality?" *New England Journal of Medicine* 317: 1674–80.

Eddy, D. 1990a. "Practice Policies—What Are They?" *Journal of the American Medical Association* 263: 877–80.

———. 1990b. "Practice Policies: Where Do They Come From?" *Journal of the American Medical Association* 263: 1265–75.

Ellwood, P. 1988. "Shattuck Lecture—Outcomes Management: A Technology of Patient Experience." *New England Journal of Medicine* 318: 1549–56.

Evans, R., and G. Stoddart. 1990. "Producing Health, Consuming Health Care." *Social Science and Medicine* 31: 1347–63.

Fowler, F., J. Wennberg, R. Timothy, M. Barry, A. Mulley, and D. Hanley. 1988. "Symptom Status and Quality of Life Following Prostatectomy." *Journal of the American Medical Association* 259: 3018–22.

Fuchs, V. 1974. *Who Shall Live?* New York: Basic Books.

Geehr, E., and R. Salluzzo. 1990. "Clinical Practice Guidelines: Promise or Illusion?" *Physician Executive* 17 (4): 13–16.

Gleicher, N. 1984. "Cesarian Section Rates in the United States: The Short-term Failure of the National Consensus Development Conference in 1980." *Journal of the American Medical Association* 252: 3273–76.

Gordis, L. 1973. Effectiveness of Comprehensive-Care Programs in Preventing Rheumatic Fever." *New England Journal of Medicine* 289: 331–35.

HDFP. 1979. "Five-year Findings of the Hypertension Detection and Follow-up Program. I. Reduction in Mortality of Persons with High Blood Pressure,

Including Mild Hypertension." *Journal of the American Medical Association* 242: 2562–71.

Hill, M., D. Levine, and P. Whelton. 1988. "Awareness, Use, and Impact of the 1984 Joint National Committee Consensus Report on High Blood Pressure." *American Journal of Public Health* 78: 1190–94.

Hollingsworth, J. R. 1981. "Inequality in Levels of Health in England and Wales, 1891–1971." *Journal of Health and Social Behavior* 22: 268–83.

Joint National Committee on Detection, Evaluation, and Treatment of High Blood Pressure. 1989. *The 1988 Report of the Joint National Committee on Detection, Evaluation, and Treatment of High Blood Pressure/National High Blood Pressure Education Program, National Heart, Lung, and Blood Institute.* NIH No. 89-1088. Bethesda, MD: National Institutes of Health.

Knowles, J. 1977. "Doing Better and Feeling Worse: Health in the United States." *Daedalus* 106 (1): 1–278.

Kosecoff, J., D. Kanouse, W. Rogers, et al. 1987. "Effects of the National Institutes of Health Consensus Development Program on Physician Practice." *Journal of the American Medical Association* 258: 2708–13.

Lalonde, M. 1975. *A New Perspective on the Health of Canadians.* Ottawa: Information Canada.

Lomas, J., G. Anderson, K. Domnick-Pierre, E. Vayda, M. Enkin, and W. Hannah. 1989. "Do Practice Guidelines Guide Practice? The Effect of a Consensus Statement on the Practice of Physicians." *New England Journal of Medicine* 321: 1306–11.

Luft, H., J. Bunker, and A. Enthoven. 1979. "Should Operations be Regionalized? The Empirical Relation between Surgical Volume and Mortality." *New England Journal of Medicine* 301: 1364–69.

Martini, C., G. J. B. Allan, J. Davison, and E. M. Backett. 1977. "Health Indexes Sensitive to Medical Care Variation." *International Journal of Health Services* 7: 293–309.

McKinlay, J., and S. McKinlay. 1977. "The Questionable Contribution of Medical Measures to the Decline of Mortality in the United States in the Twentieth Century." *Milbank Memorial Fund Quarterly* 55: 405–28.

Milio, N. 1983. *Primary Care and the Public's Health.* Lexington, MA: Lexington Books.

National Leadership Commission on Health Care. 1989. *For the Health of a Nation: A Shared Responsibility. Report of the National Leadership Commission on Health Care.* Ann Arbor: Health Administration Press.

Newhouse, J., and L. Friedlander. 1979. "The Relationship between Medical Resources and Measures of Health: Some Additional Evidence." *Journal of Human Resources* 15: 201–18.

Office of Technology Assessment. 1988. *The Quality of Medical Care: Information for Consumers.* Washington, DC: U.S. Government Printing Office.

Park, R., R. Brook, J. Kosecoff, J. Keesey, L. Rubenstein, E. Keeler, K. Kahn, W. Rogers, and M. Chassin. 1990. "Explaining Variations in Hospital Death Rates: Randomness, Severity of Illness, Quality of Care." *Journal of the American Medical Association* 264: 484–90.

Raskin, I. E., and C. W. Maklan. 1991. "Medical Treatment Effectiveness Research:

A View from Inside the Agency for Health Care Policy and Research." *Evaluation and the Health Professions* 14: 161–86.

Relman, A. 1988. "Assessment and Accountability: The Third Revolution in Medical Care." *New England Journal of Medicine* 319: 1220–22.

Stewart, A., S. Greenfield, R. Hays, K. Wells, W. Rogers, S. Berry, E. McGlynn, and J. Ware. 1989. "Functional Status and Well-being of Patients with Chronic Conditions: Results from the Medical Outcomes Study." *Journal of the American Medical Association* 262: 907–13.

Surgeon General. 1979. *Healthy People—The Surgeon General's Report on Health Promotion and Disease Prevention.* Washington, DC: U.S. Government Printing Office.

Tarlov, A., J. Ware, S. Greenfield, et al. 1989. "The Medical Outcomes Study: An Application of Methods for Monitoring the Results of Medical Care." *Journal of the American Medical Association* 262: 925–30.

VA Cooperative Study Group. 1970. "Effects of Treatment on Morbidity in Hypertension. II. Results in Patients with Diastolic Blood Pressure Averaging 90 through 114 mm Hg." *Journal of the American Medical Association* 213: 1143–52.

Valdez, R. B., R. Brook, W. Rogers, et al. 1985. "Consequences of Cost-Sharing for Children's Health." *Pediatrics* 75: 952–61.

Wennberg, J. 1984. "Dealing with Medical Practice Variations: A Proposal for Action." *Health Affairs* 3 (March): 6–32.

———. 1987. "Population Illness Rates Do Not Explain Population Hospitalization Rates—A Comment on Mark Blumberg's Thesis that Morbidity Adjusters Are Needed to Interpret Small Area Variations." *Medical Care* 25: 354–59.

———. 1990a. "Outcomes Research, Cost Containment, and the Fear of Health Care Rationing." *New England Journal of Medicine* 323: 1202–4.

———. 1990b. "Small Area Analysis and the Medical Care Outcome Problem." In *Research Methodology: Strengthening Causal Interpretations of Nonexperimental Data*, edited by L. Sechrest, B. Starfield, and J. Bunker. Rockville, MD: Agency for Health Care Policy and Research.

Wennberg, J., J. Bunker, and B. Barnes. 1980. "The Need for Assessing the Outcome of Common Medical Practices." *Annual Review of Public Health* 1: 277–95.

Wennberg, J., J. Freeman, R. Shelton, and T. Bubolz. 1989. "Hospital Use and Mortality among Medicare Beneficiaries in Boston and New Haven." *New England Journal of Medicine* 321: 1168–73.

Wennberg, J., and A. Gittelsohn. 1973. "Small Area Variations in Health Care Delivery." *Science* 182: 1102–8.

Wennberg, J., A. Mulley, D. Hanley, R. Timothy, F. Fowler, N. Roos, M. Barry, K. McPherson, E. R. Greenber, D. Soule, T. Bubolz, E. Fisher, and D. Malenka. 1988. "An Assessment of Prostatectomy for Benign Urinary Tract Obstruction: Geographic Variations and the Evaluation of Medical Care Outcomes." *Journal of the American Medical Association* 259: 3027–30.

Wennberg, J., N. Roos, L. Sola, A. Schorri, and R. Jaffe. 1987. "Use of Claims Data Systems to Evaluate Health Care Outcomes." *Journal of the American Medical Association* 257: 933–36.

Efficiency: Concepts and Methods

The fundamental questions underlying the *efficiency* of medical care are: what combination of medical care goods and services will be produced with society's limited resources, how are they produced, and are we obtaining the maximum value in terms of consumer well-being? The corollary issues are: what fundamental mechanisms are available for making these decisions, and which approach will lead to the "best" performance for a given society?

All modern societies allocate a large portion of their wealth to the provision of health care services. Growth in health care expenditures has been labeled a crisis in these countries, and efforts have focused on containment of cost increases. The United States leads the world both in terms of the level and growth of health care spending and in efforts to study the problems of access, quality, and cost of health care. In 1960, 5.3 percent of the U.S. gross national product was spent on health care; the figure was 12.2 percent in 1990 and is projected to reach 15 percent by the year 2000 (Levit et al. 1991; Office of National Cost Estimates 1990). The enormous cost and price increases in the health care system, evidence on the possible lack of effectiveness of many medical procedures, and the renewed interest in non–health care determinants of health suggest that the current allocation of resources to medical care is not efficient.

A related issue is the degree to which medical care services are produced at costs higher than the minimum possible costs, given current technology. Are resources organized and managed in a manner that minimizes the cost of production of services? Are personnel, supplies, and equipment paid for at rates that represent their cost in their next-best alternative use? Thus, the questions of how much to spend on health care, what health care services to provide, and how to provide them have become important policy issues. Because of the nature of health and health care, the status of health care as a good that many feel should be available regardless of one's ability to pay, the impingement of health care costs on public budgets, and the lack of information and other market imperfections, the solution cannot simply be left to the operation of the private market. There is a constant search for a better understanding of these problems and how the "system" operates, and for policies that will improve the access, cost, and quality of medical care.

In aggregate terms, both the efficiency and equity of the U.S. health care system compare unfavorably to Canada and several western European countries. Analysts in the United States have examined those countries both to obtain points of reference for our own problems and to gain insight into the possible solutions. Despite their relatively low expenditures and broad coverage, those countries also perceive severe problems with their health care systems and they look to the U.S. for innovative health care delivery and financing systems and especially for our extensive health services research base on the effectiveness, efficiency, and equity of alternative medical care systems and services.

Because of the concern about past and projected public and private payer budgets for health care, the policy debate has focused on cost containment rather than achieving the greatest value for the available resources. Ideally, cost containment would first be achieved by eliminating spending on services that were detrimental or had no effect on patient health status. Then, if further reductions were required, services would be ranked and funded according to their yield in health improvement per dollar. While the State of Oregon has struggled to implement a system for rationing medical care, to date, policymakers have no satisfactory mechanism for making these technically and ethically difficult decisions (Eddy 1991; Hadorn 1991).

Dating back to the Committee on the Costs of Medical Care (Falk, Rorem, and Ring 1933), analysts have documented the rising cost and related inefficiency of the U.S. medical care system. Factors contributing to cost increases have been the aging population, rapid development of medical technology, growth in third-party payment, the rising cost of malpractice and defensive medicine, and medical and general price inflation (Aaron 1991). Exacerbating these problems is the highly fragmented payment system of over 1,500 private insurers that makes it extremely difficult to control the system through regulatory measures. Beginning in the 1960s, there have been many government and private-sector efforts to stem the rising cost of medical care and achieve a more rational and fair allocation of resources. These efforts include health planning, utilization review, price controls, rate setting, increased copayments, and competition from alternative delivery systems. While there have been local successes (e.g., in Hawaii and Rochester, New York), none has succeeded on a regional or national level (Davis et al. 1990; Moon and Holahan 1992; General Accounting Office 1993).

The area of physician payment serves as an example of the efficiency problems inherent in the U.S. medical care system. Both researchers and policymakers have addressed the problem in recent years through a major new physician payment reform phased in for the Medicare program, beginning in 1992. The link between the payment system and the issue of efficiency, along with the government's proposed solution, the resource-based relative value scale (RBRVS), is explained in Chapter 5.

Chapter 4 defines the concept of efficiency, describes the regulatory and market strategies various countries have implemented to achieve it, and examines the methods used to determine the extent to which it has been achieved.

Conceptual Framework and Definitions

Efficiency

For society as a whole, efficiency requires that we produce the combination of goods and services with the highest attainable total value, given our limited resources and technology (Byrns and Stone 1987). This requires attainment of both allocative and production efficiency. Allocative efficiency depends on attainment of the "right" (most valued) mix of outputs (Davis et al. 1990). Production efficiency is producing a given level of output at minimum cost.

Allocative inefficiency may occur even in a production-efficient health system, one that produces each service at the lowest possible cost, if it produces too many or too few of some services relative to the needs and wants of society. Allocative efficiency problems arise in health care when substantial resources are allocated to treatments of questionable effectiveness while proven screening and prenatal preventive services are neglected. In a broader context, a society may obtain much greater value, and health, by diverting resources from medical care to education, job training, and community development.

Production efficiency problems occur when care is not managed in a way that maximizes potential productivity, for example, when physicians provide services that could be provided just as well by nurses or other less-expensive health personnel, and when practice does not take advantage of economies of scale, as in the production of laboratory services. These concepts of efficiency will be examined at the level of individual practitioners and hospitals and at the national health system–level.

Figure 4.1 diagrams combinations of goods and services that could be produced with society's resources during a given period of time. Within the figure, the curve AB represents the production possibility frontier; points on the curve represent maximum output possible, given current technology and the most efficient production methods. If actual production is inside the curve, as at point C, production efficiency is not being achieved. Within the shaded area, improvements in production efficiency could expand production of health care without reducing output of other goods and services, or vice versa. Once the frontier is reached, however, expansion of one commodity is at the expense of the other. Thus, allocative decisions must be made in terms of the trade-off between medical care and other goods and services.

The production possibility frontier only illustrates that alternative combinations are possible. It does not identify the allocatively efficient combination. Resource allocation is a complex, dynamic process that depends on a combination of individual choice and government tax and spending decisions. With a growing economy and technological base, the frontier is continually expanding, with technology itself being the focus of concern. The well-being of society is subject to decisions about the allocation of resources to technology and to medical care and other goods and services.

As shown in Chapter 5, examples of misallocation and inefficient production of health care can be documented. Nonetheless, the *optimal* allocation of resources and production methods is not known. Three major problems confront analysts and policymakers attempting to evaluate

Figure 4.1   Production Possibility Frontier

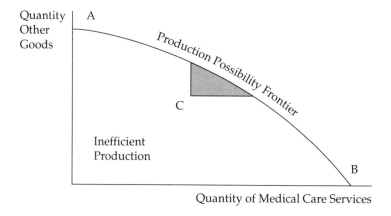

Quantity of Medical Care Services

health care resource allocation issues. The first problem is limited theoretical and empirical information on how to analyze the effects of resource allocation decisions on social well-being. Second, and related, is the problem of limited information on the relationship between medical care utilization and health. Third, both market and regulatory systems have proven to be highly imperfect mechanisms for allocating resources in the medical care sector of the economy.

Philosophers have long sought to develop theories and practical guides to define and measure social welfare. Vilfredo Pareto (1848–1923)[1] developed much of the underpinnings of welfare economics, a collection of analytic devices and concepts for evaluating resource allocation decisions. Central to this work is the Pareto optimum, which occurs when all mutually beneficial exchanges have been made such that no one person can be made better off without making someone else worse off. With freedom to trade, rational individuals or their proxies make trades that they believe benefit them and will take advantage of all opportunities to do so. However, there are many possible Pareto optimum allocations, depending on the distribution of income. Identifying and achieving the one that maximizes social well-being involves trade-offs between winners and losers and knowledge of a social welfare function.

A social welfare function describes a decision maker's preferences among alternative combinations of individual utilities (Stokey and Zeckhauser 1978). It describes how the decision maker would trade off gains in utility by some people for losses by others. For example, how is social welfare affected by allocating less to public education and more to health clinics for low-income families? To answer this question requires that we combine individual preferences to provide a ranking of welfare for society as a whole.

Arrow (1963) has demonstrated that development of such a function at the overall societal level is not possible. It has, however, been shown in theory that competitive markets can yield a Pareto optimum (Stokey and Zeckhauser 1978). Informed rational consumers make mutually beneficial trades, and competition forces producers to seek efficient methods of production and respond to consumer preferences.

Medical care, however, diverges from some fundamental properties of a perfect market. The basic conditions of a competitive market are: (1) free entry to and exit from the market by buyers and sellers, (2) many well-informed buyers and sellers, no one of whom is large enough to influence market price, and (3) no collusion among buyers and sellers, that is, they act independently. Many medical care market areas are too small to support competition, especially for services of specialists and hospitals; historically, the market has been characterized by price discrimination and collusion (Kessel 1958), ostensibly to protect consumers and provide access for those who cannot pay; asymmetry of information puts consumers at a disadvantage vis-à-vis providers; and entry by providers is strictly limited by licensing and regulation of the professions and facilities (Fuchs 1972).

In addition, Robinson and Luft (1987, 1988) have shown that under current hospital payment arrangements, greater competition leads to higher cost and lower production efficiency because hospitals compete on a nonprice basis by providing more amenities and more service capacity to attract patients and providers, respectively.

Allocative efficiency in health care depends on the contribution of medical care to the health and well-being of the population. Evans and Stoddart (1990) have suggested that medical care may at some point have a negative marginal effect on well-being due to the drain on resources that would be devoted to goods and services, such as education and housing, that may have an even greater positive effect on health. As described in Chapter 2, this raises difficult evaluation questions regarding the effect of medical care and other investments on health and well-being that we are just beginning to understand.

Given the uncertainty, complexity, and importance of medical care, societies have developed mechanisms for making resource allocation decisions. These include *need*, which primarily undergirds regulatory-based approaches, and *consumer demand*, which underlies market-based approaches.

Need

Need, as defined by health professionals (Bognanno and Bartlett 1971), has formed the basis for regulatory approaches to medical care resource allocation. Need can also be defined from a more patient-oriented perspective. Need exists when someone is better off with a treatment than without it, and the improvement is measured in terms of a person's health (Williams 1974). Therefore, unless health care professionals deem a treatment to be effective *and* the patient values its outcome, the treatment is not "needed."

While these are useful concepts for determining the care patients require, there are severe conceptual and practical problems with using this approach as a basis for resource allocation. First, there is no objective basis upon which to rank health needs and to compare them with other needs of individuals and populations. Second, needs, even with this restrictive definition, appear to be insatiable, and thus still require rationing. When some needs are met, the health care industry defines new areas not previously addressed by medicine. Third, the relationship between providing medical care services and reducing health needs is often unclear if not nonexistent (see Chapter 3 for a detailed discussion of this issue). Fourth, resources provided to meet need as defined by health professionals or government agencies may go unutilized because the population does not demand them (Feldstein 1988).

Consumer demand

Consumer demand (what consumers are willing and able to buy at alternative prices) is another important criterion for allocating resources. Need, as perceived by the consumer, is a major but not the sole determinant of demand for health care. Conceptually, consumers compare the marginal value (benefit) and marginal cost associated with alternative uses of their limited money and time resources, and make allocation decisions in their own best interest.[2]

The concept of demand is represented in Figure 4.2 as a demand curve. It shows the quantities of a good or service, e.g., routine doctor visits (horizontal axis), that an individual is willing and able to purchase at alternative prices (vertical axis) during a given period of time. Consumers are assumed to be well-informed about prices and services, and attempt to make choices that maximize their well-being. A host of factors affect the position and slope of the demand curve, including consumer income, tastes and preferences, and the prices of other related goods and services. The typical demand curve is downward sloping because (1) as price falls consumers are able to buy more, (2) the service is less costly relative to other substitute services (services that serve the same ends, e.g., outpatient and inpatient surgery for minor problems), and (3) the marginal value of the service to the consumer falls as more is consumed in a given period of time. The demand curve represents the marginal value of the service to the consumer at alternative levels of consumption (Q), and the market price (P) represents the marginal cost of the service to the consumer. By consuming at the level (Q') corresponding to that at which a given price (P') intersects the demand curve (point E), the consumer maximizes well-being. For quantities of doctor visits that exceed Q', given the price P', marginal cost is greater than marginal benefit (D), making the consumer worse off.

Market demand is merely the aggregation of the individual demands of market participants. While demand is an individual concept and depends on individual behavior, it is aggregations of individuals that form markets. Prices and quantities of goods and services are then determined by the operation of supply and demand in markets.

In a competitive market, supply represents the amount of a good or service that suppliers are willing to sell at alternative prices during a given period of time (Figure 4.3). The curve is positive or upward

Figure 4.2   Individual Demand Curve

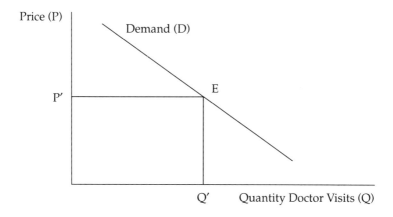

sloping, meaning that greater quantities are supplied at higher prices. The position of the supply curve depends on technology (the ability to transform inputs into output), the prices of inputs such as wages and rents, and the objectives of suppliers, i.e., whether they are attempting to maximize profits or services or some combination. For example, technological innovation in electronics has markedly increased productivity and allowed producers to offer the same products at lower prices, a rightward shift in the supply curve. Similarly, increases in wages and other input costs would require higher prices for the same number of units, resulting in a leftward shift in the supply curve. Market supply is the aggregation of individual supply of market participants.

The intersection of market supply and demand determines the equilibrium (E), market price (P′), and quantity of services (Q′) for a given period of time (Figure 4.4). This is the model that undergirds the market approach to health care reform. As any model, it is a simplification of reality, and any application must deal with the disparities between it and the real world of health care. But consumer choice and self-regulating market forces are assumed in such a model.

By rapidly adjusting to changes in consumer preferences, incomes, resource scarcity, and technology, competitive markets generally provide a flexible mechanism for solving the basic economic problems of what is produced, how it is produced, and for whom. For many goods, and possibly for routine medical care, consumers appear to be the best judge of their needs and desires relative to other uses of their resources.[3] Under competitive market conditions, producers who fail to respond

Figure 4.3   Individual Supply Curve

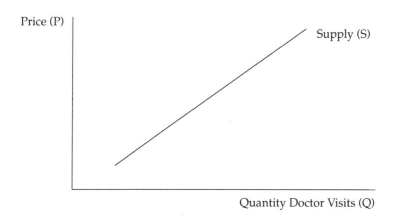

Figure 4.4   Market Demand and Supply

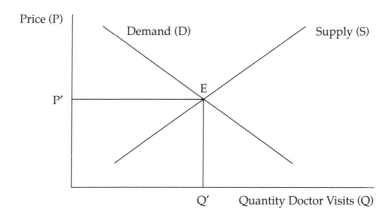

to consumer demand, charge prices above the market rate, or use inefficient production methods are forced out of business, and consumers individually allocate resources to maximize their well-being, leading the system toward a Pareto optimum allocation of resources.

As indicated earlier, this model does not fully apply to medical care because of several inherent market limitations. There are significant externalities (instances in which one person's consumption or production affects another person's well-being). For example, a person who obtains immunizations to prevent infectious diseases provide benefits to others by reducing their risk of contracting the disease. Private markets tend to underinvest in these types of services because benefits to third parties are not directly incorporated in market demand by those who seek services. Similarly, people seem to care that others have access to basic medical care, and therefore benefit when others gain access to care who would otherwise not obtain it. Markets alone have no mechanism for translating this value into the desired result.

Another problem with a private medical care market is the lack of independence between demand and supply, so-called supplier-induced demand. Provider interests may affect consumer demand due to the large disparity of information between provider and consumer and the fact that a third party often pays for a substantial portion of services rendered (Reinhardt 1987). Thus, the provider, who is generally not financially disinterested, has a major influence over consumer demand, greatly diminishing the independent role of consumer choice in the market for medical care services. Due to these problems, as well as other monopoly elements such as the lack of free entry and exit to the industry by producers, price collusion among producers, and the fact that the available distribution of income may exclude some groups from medical care, the market fails to achieve satisfactory allocation and distribution of medical care resources.

All modern societies appear to accept the limitations of private markets and regulatory strategies for achieving efficiency. The problem is how to balance and coordinate the respective roles of government and private forces. Governments become directly involved in the financing and provision of medical care services to their populations. The degree of involvement varies from direct provision of most services to providing coverage for the most vulnerable populations within the context of a largely private medical care system. Given these problems, countries have selected different mechanisms for making medical care resource allocation decisions. These will be illustrated by reference to the United States and other Western countries and how they are positioned along a continuum of the degree to which decisions are governed by market forces.

Role of incentives and controls

Market continuum

Anderson (1989, 19) has noted that countries in the developed world vary along a continuum of market-minimized (left) to market-maximized (right), in the organization and financing of their medical care sectors:

The more one agrees with the position toward the right end of the continuum, the more likely one is to favor private insurance that covers all sorts of contingencies, including unexpected costs of personal health services. As one approaches the position toward the left end of the continuum, one eventually subscribes to a health service completely owned, financed, and salaried by the state and paid for out of general revenue.

On the right-hand side of the continuum, one is likely to believe in cash indemnity for health services and financial controls on patients. This view regards providers of services as essentially autonomous sellers of services; patients, as it were, hire a physician to manage their service needs. On the left-hand side of the continuum, with the highly structured and completely government-owned health service, there would be no charge to the patient at the time of service. Charges to the patient at that time, no matter how small they were, would be regarded as an undesirable barrier to access to services for prevention, early diagnosis, and treatment. At the right-hand extreme, patients are assumed to know their self-interest well enough not to be inhibited by charges at the time of service.

Table 4.1 provides data on the role of the public sector in the provision of health insurance coverage and payment for medical care services by country. The United Kingdom has traditionally represented the market-minimized extreme with a national health service, government ownership of hospitals, direct employment of hospital physicians, nurses, and allied health workers, and central budgetary control. The market-maximized extreme is represented by the United States, with a majority of private hospitals, private physicians and other health workers, private insurance covering a majority of the population, out-of-pocket payment representing 20 percent of expenditures, and a plethora of payers without coordination of payment. In between, but leaning more toward the market-minimized side are the Scandinavian countries and France. Countries leaning more toward market mechanisms, although far left of the United States, are Australia, Canada, Germany, Switzerland, and Japan.

While all countries seek to achieve equity, efficiency, and overall cost control in their health sectors, each country has a unique approach to addressing these basic economic and social issues. The market-minimized systems tend to rely more on direct government or quasi-government controls to achieve the desired results, while the market-maximized approach is to rely on the private market to allocate resources and use the government to provide for the most vulnerable segments of the population. The weight of the evidence suggests that the United States, with its market-based system, has failed to achieve equity or cost control, and may be less efficient in terms of health outcomes achieved for the investment (Organization for Economic Cooperation and Development 1987).

Table 4.1   Public Coverage against Cost of Medical Care and Average Percentage of Bill Paid by Public Insurance: Selected Countries, 1990

	Percentage of Population with Public Coverage		Percentage of Costs Paid by Public Insurance	
Country	*Hospital Care*	*Ambulatory Care*	*Hospital Care*	*Ambulatory Care*
United Kingdom	100	100	99	88
Finland	100	100	82	72
Norway	100	100	100	—
Sweden	100	100	100	90
France	99	98	91	60
Australia	100	100	78	58
Canada	100	100	91	72
Germany	92	92	98	92
Switzerland	100	100	100	79
Japan	100	100	93	85
United States	44	44	55	56

Source: OECD Health Data 1991.

On the plus side, U.S. patients may benefit from rapid technological advancement and diffusion, innovative delivery and financing systems, and advances in research on medical care effectiveness (Enthoven 1990). Each country's approach to health care may depend largely on its culture, history, and political situation. While nations can use others' experience as a point of reference for their own performance and gain ideas for application at home, there is no clear model that is universally efficient (Swint 1990).

Management continuum

An important difference between the market-oriented system in the United States and the systems in other developed countries lies in the approach to controlling cost and resource allocation. The U.S. approach has been characterized as micromanagement as contrasted with the macromanagement practiced in other countries (Reinhardt 1990). Micromanagement tends to rely on incentives such as copayments for consumers and capitation payment for providers in competing health plans, whereas macromanagement relies on controls such as fee schedules, global budgets, and limits on diffusion of technology to achieve health system objectives.

Since the market-based U.S. payment and delivery system is so decentralized, emphasis is put on affecting the behavior of individual providers and patients with a mix of incentives and controls. Thus, there are elaborate methods for utilization review, individual fee screens, selective contracting, capitated payment for providers, and now practice guidelines. For patients, there are deductibles, coinsurance, limits on coverage, queues for appointments, limits on provider choice, and requirements to participate in utilization review procedures. Competition is introduced through an array of health plan choices for those with public or private insurance.

One result of micromanagement is very high administrative costs: one estimate shows them at 24 percent of health care costs in the United States versus 11 percent in Canada (Woolhandler and Himmelstein 1991). In Canada and Europe, administration is simplified by having one or few sources of payment and sets of rules. With global hospital budgets and fixed fee schedules, there is little need for close monitoring of provider behavior. The key to macromanagement is limiting the sources of payment and controlling the amount to be paid. This includes regional planning to limit the physical facilities and assure fair distribution, thereby providing the constraints within which providers work. The system results in queues for expensive, high-technology procedures and equipment, forcing physicians to allocate services based on the urgency of the cases. Evans (1986, 602) has characterized the basic attitudes of providers in the United States and Canada toward the use of resources and procedures as, "when in doubt do versus when in doubt don't."

Payment methods. Alternative methods of paying physicians and hospitals provide different incentives regarding efficiency (D'Intignano 1990). The United States has many different payment methods and sources operating simultaneously, while other countries have a primary method for hospital and physician reimbursement and funnel payment through very few channels, compared to the plethora of payment sources in the United States (Reinhardt 1990). For example, physicians in the United States are paid by local, state, and federal agencies, by over 1,500 insurers, and by direct out-of-pocket payments from patients. Methods of payment include fee-for-service, salary, and capitation, none of which is strictly limited by regulation. Fee-for-service based on usual and customary fees has dominated, and while it provides an incentive for high productivity, it also leads to inflation and a proliferation of procedures with low marginal value relative to cost (Moloney and Rogers 1979).

Canada and Germany have also relied on fee-for-service payment of physicians, but fees are strictly controlled. To address the problem of volume expansion, Germany has developed a system of global prospective fees. The fee system specifies a relative value for each service. The monetary value of each relative value point is determined retrospectively by dividing a global physician budget by the total number of relative value points (the product of number of services and relative value per service) billed by the physicians during a period. The budget is allowed to grow only at the rate of growth of income in the economy. Thus, if volume expands too much, price per unit is reduced to keep total expenditures within the growth limit. This method has allowed Germany to stabilize health care expenditures as a percentage of gross domestic product (GDP).

Per diem prices, global budgets, prospective payment by diagnosis-related groups, and prepayment are major methods for paying for hospital services. Each method provides different financial incentives for the hospital and has different implications for efficiency (Dowling 1974). In the pluralistic U.S. system, each method is being used, although traditionally hospitals have been paid per diem rates plus fees for individual ancillary services. These prices were based on costs, although cross-subsidization of patients and services was widespread until payers cracked down on this practice and competition expanded.

Again, the federal Medicare program has led the way in reforming hospital payment, implementing the prospective payment system in 1983. PPS was designed to pay a fixed amount per episode of hospital care defined by one of 483 diagnostic groups. It provided an incentive for hospitals to encourage doctors to reduce length of stay and to provide hospital services more efficiently, because each hospital could retain any surplus in payments over costs. Peer review organizations were to monitor the necessity of admissions and the adequacy of care, to offset the incentive to admit more patients, underserve, and discharge too soon.

While extremely difficult to demonstrate conclusively, PPS has generally been judged successful in containing hospital costs under Medicare without harming patients (Kahn et al. 1990; Russell 1989). However, one result of PPS was rapid expansion in outpatient hospital services, home care, and long-term care. This may be partially remedied by a new proposal to bundle outpatient hospital services into 297 ambulatory groups for each of which the government would pay a standard amount (Pear 1991). While hospitals profited initially under PPS, subsequent restrictions on payment increases have left them with current operating margins near zero (Aaron 1991; American Hospital Association 1993). Schwartz and Mendelson (1991) have shown that hospital cost-containment strategies in the 1980s, including PPS, did not affect the underlying increase in hospital costs in the United States. Reductions in the rate of growth in Medicare expenditure were offset by an increase in non-Medicare spending.

Planning and fee controls. Canada has global hospital budgets and regional health planning to control the cost of hospital care and the diffusion of medical technology. In Germany, hospitals are financed through all-inclusive per diems negotiated between hospitals and the regional associations of sickness funds (Jonsson 1990). Rates are subject to approval by the state which also approves and pays for capital spending, based on statewide hospital planning. Relative to the United States, the Canadian system has high utilization of inpatient days and constraints on high-cost surgical and diagnostic procedures. The system suffers from the "bed blocker" phenomenon. Older individuals whose condition does not require the high intensity of care available in hospitals, have lengths of stay on the order of 50 to 60 days. Germany appears to have a similar experience, with even higher inpatient utilization rates (see Table 4.2). Hospital bed days per person per year have declined in the United States from 2.3 in 1970 to 1.3 in 1989, while Canada has remained constant at around 2.0 and Germany has been stable at about 3.5. Average length of stay has also declined in the United States since 1970. In Germany, the average fell from 24.9 in 1970 to 16.2 in 1989, in contrast to Canada, where there was an increase from 11.5 in 1970 to 13.2 in 1987.

Spending constraints have resulted in queues in Canada. For example, in Ontario during the fall of 1990, at least 90 percent of programs providing computerized axial tomography (CAT) scans, magnetic resonance imaging (MRI), cardiovascular surgery, eye surgery, orthopedic surgery, and lithotripsy reported queues for elective cases, and at least 30 percent of the programs reported queues for urgent cases ("involving serious medical conditions"). Only the MRI and lithotripsy programs reported queues for emergent ("life-threatening") cases, however (General Accounting Office 1991).

Although all three countries have experienced a compound annual growth in per capita health care expenditure on the order of 10 percent per year, both Canada and Germany have been more successful in controlling health care costs than the United States. From 1970 to 1990, the percent of GDP spent on health care rose from 7.4 to 12.4 in the United States compared to an increase from 7.1 to 9.0 in Canada and from 5.9 to 8.1 in Germany. For the same period, per capita health care spending increased from $346 to $2,566 in the United States compared to increases from $279 to $1,933 in Canada and from $179 to $1,899 in Germany. Similar patterns prevail for hospital care (see Table 4.3).

The key to cost control in these macromanaged systems is having a dominant source of payment that fixes the budget for a given period of time. Growth in the budget is generally limited by growth in the economy. Thus, the Canadian and German systems rely on control of the funds available to physician and hospital providers rather than on the

Table 4.2 Use of Inpatient Health Care: Selected Countries, 1970–89

Year	Hospital Bed Days/ Person per Year			Hospital Admission Rates (Percentage of Population) per Year			Average Length of Stay in Inpatient Institutions			Consultations and Visits per Capita		
	U.S.	Canada	Germany	U.S.	Canada	Germany	U.S.	Canada	Germany	U.S.	Canada	Germany
1970	2.3	2.0	3.6	15.5	16.5	15.4	14.9	11.5	24.9	4.6	—	—
1975	1.9	2.0	3.6	16.7	16.6	16.9	11.4	11.2	22.2	5.1	4.9	10.9
1980	1.7	2.1	3.6	17.1	15.1	18.8	10.0	12.9	19.7	4.8	5.4	11.5
1985	1.4	2.1	3.5	15.2	14.8	19.9	9.2	13.4	18.0	5.2	6.2	—
1987	1.3	2.1	3.5	14.1	14.7	21.1	9.3	13.2	17.1	5.3	6.6	—
1989	1.3	2.0	3.4	13.7	—	21.5	—	—	16.2	5.3	—	—

Source: OECD Health Data 1991.

Table 4.3   Health Care Expenditures: Selected Countries, 1970–90

Year	Health Care Expenditures as Percentage of GDP			Health Care Expenditures per Capita, in U.S. $			Inpatient Expenditures per Capita, in U.S. $		
	U.S.	Canada	Germany	U.S.	Canada	Germany	U.S.	Canada	Germany
1970	7.4	7.1	5.9	346	279	179	153	146	64
1975	8.4	7.2	8.1	592	529	549	277	286	208
1980	9.3	7.4	8.4	1,063	806	1,106	520	424	399
1985	10.7	8.5	8.7	1,711	1,171	883	819	594	324
1990	12.4	9.0	8.1	2,566	1,933	1,899	1,191	—	—

Source: OECD Health Data 1991.

mixture of market incentives and controls present in the United States. Because of the Canadian and German track records, many argue that the United States would be wise to pursue a similar system of macrocontrol and abandon attempts to develop an efficient system based on market concepts (General Accounting Office 1991). While global budgets may reduce spending, they do not necessarily lead to either greater allocative efficiency or greater production efficiency. In the process of controlling total costs, perverse incentives may be created for both allocation and production. Hospitals may pressure physicians to keep beds full to justify continuation or expansion of the hospital budget. More-efficient, innovative outpatient delivery may lag because of the lack of incentives to develop new services.

Managed competition. Enthoven and Kronick (1989) have proposed the development of managed competition as a method for allocating medical care resources and controlling costs within the context of a market-based system. This approach depends on market incentives to motivate health plans and providers to be efficient and responsive to consumer needs and demands. Employers (private sponsors) and state government agencies (public sponsors) of health benefits would aggressively monitor and manage competition among health plans in the health care market. Employers would play their traditional role in health benefits, and a public agency or agencies designated by the state would serve as a broker for self-employed and other persons who choose to obtain health insurance through the state sponsor. Fixed contributions (with a limit on tax deductibility) from sponsors would provide incentives for cost-conscious choice by consumers. Pieces of this approach have been implemented to varying degrees, especially during the 1980s. Competing health plans, health maintenance organizations, preferred provider organizations, point-of-service plans, and plans with exclusive provider arrangements have experienced rapid growth, enrolling between 50 million and 60 million persons at the beginning of 1990, including 35 million in 591 HMOs (Health Insurance Association of America 1990). Medicare developed a risk-contracting system and now enrolls one million persons in HMOs and other alternative delivery systems. The Medicaid programs in several states have changed to competitive bidding and limited choice for eligible populations (Freund et al. 1989). HMO Medicaid enrollment increased from 282,000 people in 1981 to 947,000 people in 1987.

Critics contend that efforts to control costs through health care competition have failed. Costs were not contained, and employers have not achieved savings from this strategy. Greater competition has been associated with higher costs (Robinson and Luft 1985, 1987, 1988). Aaron (1991) argues that incremental changes such as increasing competition will not solve the problem because they do not address the fundamental causes of cost inflation: the rapid development of new methods of treatment and diagnosis. Countervailing evidence is provided by the experience in California following the 1982 introduction of legislation that allowed selective contracting (Zwanziger and Melnick 1988). High hospital costs were associated with greater hospital competition prior to the introduction of the procompetition legislation. Afterwards, as predicted, hospitals in more competitive markets experienced lower costs. Enthoven and Kronick (1989) claim that real price competition has not been implemented. Employers and government either have not offered multiple choices of plans, have subsidized nearly the full price of the traditional fee-for-service plan, or have not permitted employees and beneficiaries to keep the savings from choosing less expensive plans. The result has often been adverse selection of high-risk employees into the traditional plans, with the accompanying rise in premiums and shadow pricing (pricing below but near the competition) by the competing HMO health plans. Thus, competition may have contributed to rising costs, not because price competition cannot work in medical care, but because it has not been properly implemented and managed.

Health care reform was a major issue in the recent presidential election in the United States. While committed to fundamental reform, President Clinton and the Democratic Party assessed the alternatives during the early months of the new administration. Prominent contenders were a single-payer, Canadian-style system and managed competition with expenditure limits. There are strong positions and proponents on each side of the debate, and there is no way to resolve this dispute empirically, short of implementing and evaluating a well-designed competitive plan on a state, regional, or national basis. Opponents of competition claim that social regulation has been proven in Canada and Europe and that a competitive demonstration would simply delay the inevitable and be a costly exercise. Proponents argue that a governmental solution is antithetical to the American preference for limited government and continue to affirm the theoretical efficiency of markets for resource allocation. Further, proponents contend that once a government system is established, it will be politically difficult to change, whereas if the market approach is deemed to have failed, then the nonmarket approach can be tried.

Both macro and micro health care policy and management alternatives can be examined with economic models and methods. Following is a description of selected methods and how they are applied to medical care issues.

Key Methods of Assessing the Efficiency of Medical Care

Micro level

Economists have developed a comprehensive theoretical model of production cost and efficiency. It is a normative model, expressing how the total, average, and marginal costs of a given product or commodity change under a given set of assumptions regarding the relationship between inputs and outputs (the production function), the cost of inputs, and technology. For example, inputs for ambulatory medical care may include nurse and physician time, and outputs may be defined in terms of services rendered or their effect on the health of patients. Input costs include nurse and physician earnings, rents, and the cost of supplies. Technology is defined broadly as the information and techniques required to transform inputs into outputs. The cost functions represent the minimum costs attainable for alternative combinations of inputs and the size of the production units.

Under usual assumptions, it is possible to determine the cost-minimizing mix of inputs for any level of output and the cost-minimizing size of the production unit (Byrns and Stone 1987). Even when producers have the "right" combination of inputs and size, they may fail to achieve maximum output. This may be due to poor management, low employee motivation, or other unspecified production problems and is referred to as x-inefficiency (Leibenstein 1966). X-inefficiency occurs whenever a firm produces less than the maximum possible output from given resources. Conceptually, production and cost functions can be applied to any production process, although they are less precise in areas where output is difficult to define and measure. The production and cost models have been applied to physician, hospital, and insurance services to determine the extent to which production efficiency has been achieved and how it may be enhanced. Summaries of selected studies are provided in Chapter 5.

Other efficiency analysis methods frequently applied in medical care are cost-effectiveness analysis (CEA) and cost-benefit analysis (CBA) (Drummond, Stoddart, and Torrance 1987). CEA is a systematic analysis of the effects and costs of alternative methods or programs for achieving the same objective, e.g., saving lives, preventing disease, or providing services. CEA is used when the concern is with determining production efficiency. Effects are measured in nonmonetary units.

CBA is a systematic analysis of one or more methods or programs for achieving a given objective and measures both benefits and costs in monetary units. CBA can determine whether a program is worth doing, in the sense that its benefits are greater than its costs (allocative efficiency), while CEA compares the cost of alternatives in achieving a common objective (production efficiency) without determining whether the objective itself is worth achieving. For example, what are the costs and associated savings of annual screening and treatment for diabetic retinopathy for persons in the United States? A positive net benefit indicates allocative efficiency. Society is made worse off by adopting projects whose costs outweigh benefits and better off by adopting projects whose benefits outweigh costs. While it is not practical to rank all possible competing uses of resources to achieve the optimal resource allocation, projects can be considered on an incremental basis.

CEA can be used as both a complement to and substitute for CBA. For example, to evaluate the retinopathy program, one would first determine the most efficient way to screen for the problem, given several available technologies. These production efficiency results would then feed into the CBA to address the allocation question, i.e., how much, if any, should society invest in screening and treating diabetic retinopathy? Alternatively, it may be determined that the program would not have net economic benefits because of the population affected, but may yield health benefits and should be compared with other programs in terms of cost per quality-adjusted life-year gained. Effectiveness can then be measured in terms of increases in QALY, and compared to other activities on the basis of cost per QALY. Thus, instead of monetary values, life-years are valued (quality-adjusted) according to utility values or how people feel about time spent in alternative health states ranging from states they feel would be worse than death to being completely healthy (Torrance, Boyle, and Horwood 1982). For example, while being completely healthy may be assigned a utility value of 1, the condition of blindness may be assigned a value of 0.6. If an otherwise healthy person could avert blindness for one year the gain would be 0.4 QALYs.

Use of CBA and CEA has expanded in recent years as government and industry have sought to control deficits while meeting service and production objectives. CBA was first introduced to evaluate the economic effect of public investments (Warner and Luce 1982). Expanded government funding of medical effectiveness, outcomes research, and clinical guidelines (Agency for Health Care Policy and Research 1991) provides information to carry out further economic evaluation of health care services. AHCPR has established patient outcome research teams to carry out broad investigations of alternative services or procedures for managing specific clinical conditions (see Chapter 3).

Effectiveness information can feed into new policy models designed to integrate issues of quality of life, patient functional status, and costs. Kaplan and Anderson (1988) have developed a measure that integrates the health benefit and utility frameworks for the evaluation of health care programs. Specifically, their measure integrates point-in-time estimates of function, transition among functional levels over time, utilities of health states, and mortality. It has been applied to several prevention and treatment program evaluations. Policymakers, as exemplified by the Oregon program, are beginning to apply this type of thinking, if not the exact methods, to the allocation of scarce health resources. The Oregon program attempted to rank health services according to their potential benefits, with services being limited by the total budget that is politically allocated. In this way more persons could obtain basic coverage, but some services judged to be of less value would not be covered (Eddy 1991). The federal government refused to grant a waiver to implement the Oregon program because it violated the Americans with Disabilities Act. A revised plan was approved by the Clinton administration.

Paul Feldstein (1988) has used a qualitative method for evaluating the allocative efficiency of the medical care sector. The value structure of consumer sovereignty and the criterion of maximum consumer well-being form the basis of his economic evaluation. The various sectors (e.g., insurance, hospital care, physician care) are examined in terms of the degree to which observed behavior is consistent with predictions derived from the basic economic model of the competitive market. For example, do producers strive to minimize the cost of production, and are the mix and quality of goods and services guided by consumer choices? When inconsistencies occur, the basic assumptions of the competitive model are re-examined and altered in an attempt to better explain observed behavior. Feldstein finds distortions in the insurance and health care markets that have led to misallocation of resources and inefficient production methods. These problems can be addressed through market reform, a process begun but not completed in the 1980s.

Williams (1990) has contrasted that view with a public-sector political framework that is also concerned with production efficiency. However, in this framework, allocative efficiency is judged by the electorate in terms of the extent to which the medical care system improves the health status of the population in relation to the resources allocated to it, and priorities are determined by social judgments of need. This system of resource allocation is exemplified by the reformed National Health Service in Britain. Culyer, Maynard, and Posnett (1990, 1) have summarized elements of this reform:

> The principle which permeates all these changes is the separation of the purchaser and provider functions and the creation thereby of greater "transparency" in trading so that the prices, volumes and quality of services are explicit and providers can be made more accountable. Underlying this is another principle: to create a situation in which need is better assessed at the community level with the delivery of care responding to this expressed need more efficiently.

Reform of the British system was introduced in 1989 and affects three basic elements of the National Health Service: hospital service, general practice, and community care. Large group practices and district general managers become budget holders under the reformed system. They purchase diagnostic and therapeutic services from competing public and private providers. The budget holders are responsible for assessing the health needs of their community, prioritizing those needs, and meeting them in the most cost-effective way using providers within or outside their district. Budgets are determined by a population formula weighted by need. Thus, the new market operates only on the supply side, with demand being determined not by what people are willing and able to pay but by administrative estimates of need.

The U.S. federal government recently implemented the resource-based relative value fee scale for physician services to complement the prospective payment DRG-based fee system for hospitals. In addition, work continues on medical effectiveness studies that will yield practice guidelines. These changes, wrought by government, will have profound effects on the payment for and practice of medicine in the market-oriented U.S. medical care system. These administered price systems may represent an important element in a future, macromanaged U.S. medical care system. What remains is the application of these systems to all payers under a global budget. Without expenditure caps and concentration of payment channels, the new systems represent another set of incentives or constraints faced by health care providers in a micro-managed system.

Neither evaluation, the market or the political, is more than a very rough approximation of how well the medical care system is functioning. Each represents an extremely different orientation, with the former leading to the market-maximized and the latter to the market-minimized end of the health care policy continuum. Developed Western countries use elements of each to gauge their medical care systems. Ironically, of the two countries at opposite ends of the market continuum, Britain is now introducing more consumer choice into its public system while the United States continues to expand regulation in response to political pressure to cover more of its population and control costs.

Macro level

Investigators have attempted to gain a perspective on medical care systems by comparing them to systems in other politically and economically similar countries. While there are major problems with comparisons at the system level, such as measurement of health outcomes, cultural and demographic differences, and data comparability, such comparisons do serve to raise questions about the efficiency and equity of health systems and stimulate inquiry into reasons for major observed differences (Schieber and Poullier 1990).

Researchers at the Organization for Economic Cooperation and Development (OECD) have collected data and attempted to develop standardized international health accounts for the organization's 24 member countries (Schieber and Poullier 1990). Because it is not possible to measure health outcomes in ways that are very sensitive to health care inputs (this point is elaborated in Chapter 2), these comparisons rely on aggregate measures of life expectancy, infant mortality, and cause-of-death-specific mortality. Additionally, problems of measuring efficiency are compounded by the difficulty of allocating overhead in complex multiproduct firms such as hospitals and multispecialty group practices. Comparisons thus focus on aggregate measures of input, such as numbers of doctors, nurses, hospital beds, and on intermediate outputs, such as physician visits and hospital admissions. After documenting the fact that U.S. hospitals use much more high-cost technology, more intense and costly care per hospital day, and lower lengths of stay compared to Canada and Western European countries, Aaron (1991, 86) summarized the difficulty of interpreting the data:

> Analysts remain unsure about how much of the international differences are explained by variations in intensity of service or price, or by such other factors as age composition or efficiency in the health care system. Sorting out quality-improving, but cost-increasing, variations in technology from simple price changes is a difficult task at best and sometimes impossible because prices for many kinds of health care do not exist in some countries.

The main objective of this chapter was to explain the major concepts and methods used to assess the efficiency of the medical care system: allocative and production efficiency. Allocative efficiency concerns attainment of the highest total value from the limited resources that society has available during any given period of time. This requires that a society choose the "right" most-valued mix of goods and services and that they be produced at minimum cost (maximize production efficiency).

While always imperfect in practice, analysts have developed both micro and macro approaches to efficiency assessment. Micro methods include the normative microeconomic theories of markets, including production and cost functions as applied to medical care. Also, the techniques of cost-benefit and cost-effectiveness analysis are used to examine the efficiency of production methods and resource allocation to specific health services and programs. Extensive data on the OECD countries have permitted rough comparisons between countries at the macro level in terms of spending, utilization, and health indicators for the population.

Although evaluation is difficult and limited by the complexities and uncertainties of medical care, numerous studies of efficiency have been conducted in the United States and other countries. Chapter 5 provides a selected summary of evidence on the efficiency of the U.S. medical care system.

Notes

1. For a detailed explanation of Pareto's work, see Kohler (1990), pp. 484–519.
2. "Marginal" refers to the next unit of a good or service that the consumer is considering. This differs from the average total value of all units consumed. A "rational" consumer would not purchase the next unit of a good or service if he or she perceived the benefit of that next unit to be less than the cost of the unit.
3. Even for sophisticated tertiary care, doctors have long acknowledged, if not always fostered, the patient's right to be part of the decision-making team when alternative courses of action that include alternative levels of risk, benefit, and costs are contemplated. Patient values are now being fully integrated with clinical information in patient outcome studies (Barry et al. 1988).

References

Aaron, H. 1991. *Serious and Unstable Condition: Financing America's Health Care.* Washington, DC: Brookings Institution.
Agency for Health Care Policy and Research. 1991. *Report to Congress: Progress of*

Research on Outcomes of Health Care Services and Procedures. AHCPR Pub. No. 91-0004. Rockville, MD: Agency for Health Care Policy and Research.

American Hospital Association. 1993. *Economic Trends* 8 (4):11.

Anderson, O. W. 1989. *The Health Services Continuum in Democratic States.* Ann Arbor: Health Administration Press.

Arrow, K. J. 1963. *Social Choice and Individual Values.* New Haven: Yale University Press.

Barry, M., A. Mulley, F. Fowler, and J. Wennberg. 1988. "Watchful Waiting vs. Immediate Transurethral Resection for Symptomatic Prostatism: The Importance of Patients' Preferences." *Journal of the American Medical Association* 259: 3010–17.

Bognanno, M. F., and J. C. Bartlett. 1971. "On the Demand versus Need for Medical Services and the Concept of Shortage." *American Journal of Public Health* 61: 46–64.

Byrns, R. T., and G. W. Stone. 1987. *Economics.* Glenview, IL: Scott, Foresman and Co.

Culyer, A. J., A. Maynard, and J. Posnett. 1990. "Reforming Health Care: An Introduction to the Economic Issues." In *Competition in Health Care: Reforming the NHS,* edited by A. J. Culyer, A. K. Maynard, and J. W. Posnett, 1–11. London: Macmillan Press.

Davis, K., G. F. Anderson, D. Rowland, and E. P. Steinberg. 1990. *Health Care Cost Containment.* Baltimore and London: Johns Hopkins University Press.

D'Intignano, B. M. 1990. "Incentives in Health Care Management." 2nd World Congress on Health Economics, Zurich, Switzerland.

Dowling, W. 1974. "Prospective Reimbursement of Hospitals." *Inquiry* 11: 163–80.

Drummond, M. F., G. L. Stoddart, and G. W. Torrance. 1987. *Methods for Economic Evaluation of Health Care Programmes.* Oxford: Oxford University Press.

Eddy, D. 1991. "Clinical Decision Making: From Theory to Practice—What's Going On in Oregon?" *Journal of the American Medical Association* 266: 417–20.

Enthoven, A. 1990. "What can Europeans Learn from Americans?" In *Health Care Systems in Transition,* 51–71. Paris: Organization for Economic Cooperation and Development.

Enthoven, A., and R. Kronick. 1989. "A Consumer-Choice Health Plan for the 1990s: Universal Health Insurance in a System Designed to Promote Quality and Economy." *New England Journal of Medicine* 320: 29–37.

Evans, R. 1986. "Finding the Levers, Finding the Courage: Lessons from Cost Containment in North America." *Journal of Health Politics, Policy and Law* 11: 585–614.

Evans, R., and G. Stoddart. 1990. "Producing Health, Consuming Health Care." *Social Science and Medicine* 31: 1347–63.

Falk, I. S., C. R. Rorem, and M. D. Ring. 1933. *The Cost of Medical Care.* Chicago: University of Chicago Press.

Feldstein, P. J. 1988. *Health Care Economics.* New York: John Wiley & Sons.

Freund, D., L. Rossiter, P. Fox, J. Meyer, R. Hurley, T. Carey, and J. Paul. 1989. "Evaluation of the Medicaid Competition Demonstrations." *Health Care Financing Review* 11 (2): 81–97.

96 Evaluating the Medical Care System

Fuchs, V. 1972. "Health Care and the United States Economic System: An Essay in Abnormal Physiology." *Milbank Memorial Fund Quarterly* 50: 211–37.

General Accounting Office. 1991. *Canadian Health Insurance: Lessons for the United States.* GAO/HRD-91-90. Washington, DC: U.S. General Accounting Office.

———. 1993. *Health Care: Rochester's Community Approach Yields Better Access, Lower Costs.* GAO/HRD-93-44. Washington, DC: U.S. General Accounting Office.

Hadorn, D. 1991. "Setting Health Care Priorities in Oregon: Cost-Effectiveness Meets the Rule of Rescue." *Journal of the American Medical Association* 265: 2218–25.

Health Insurance Association of America. 1990. *Source Book of Health Insurance Data.* Washington, DC: Health Insurance Association of America.

Jonsson, B. 1990. "What Can Americans Learn from Europeans?" In *Health Care Systems in Transition.* Paris: Organization for Economic Cooperation and Development.

Kahn, K. L., L. V. Rubenstein, D. Draper, J. Kosecoff, W. H. Rogers, E. B. Keeler, and R. H. Brook. 1990. "Comparing Outcomes of Care Before and After Implementation of the DRG-based Prospective Payment System." *Journal of the American Medical Association* 264: 1984–88.

Kaplan, R. M., and J. P. Anderson. 1988. "A General Health Policy Model: Update and Applications." *Health Services Research* 23: 203–35.

Kessel, R. 1958. "Price Discrimination in Medicine." *Journal of Law and Economics* 1 (1): 20–53.

Kohler, H. 1990. *Intermediate Microeconomics,* 3rd ed. Glenview, IL: Scott, Foresman and Co.

Leibenstein, H. 1966. "Allocative Efficiency vs. 'X-Efficiency'." *American Economic Review* 56: 392–415.

Levit, K. R., H. C. Lazenby, C. A. Cowan, and S. W. Letsch. 1991. "National Health Expenditures 1990." *Health Care Financing Review* 13 (1): 29–54.

Moloney, T. W., and D. E. Rogers. 1979. "Medical Technology—A Different View of the Contentious Debate over Costs." *New England Journal of Medicine* 301: 1413–19.

Moon, M., and J. Holahan. 1992. "Can States Take the Lead in Health Care Reform?" *Journal of the American Medical Association* 268: 1588–94.

OECD Health Data: A Software Package for the International Comparison of Health Care Systems. 1991. Ver. 1.01. Paris: Organization for Economic Cooperation and Development.

Office of National Cost Estimates. 1990. "National Health Expenditures 1988." *Health Care Financing Review* 11 (4): 1–41.

Organization for Economic Cooperation and Development. 1987. *Financing and Delivering Health Care.* SPS No. 4. Paris: Organization for Economic Cooperation and Development.

Pear, R. 1991. "Government Seeks New Cost Control on Medicare Plan." *New York Times,* 9 June: 1, 14.

Reinhardt, U. E. 1987. "A Clarification of Theories and Evidence on Supplier-

Induced Demand for Physicians' Services." *Journal of Human Resources* 22: 621–23.

———. 1990. "What Can Americans Learn from Europeans?" In *Health Care Systems in Transition*, 105–12. Paris: Organization for Economic Cooperation and Development.

Robinson, J. C., and H. F. Luft. 1985. "The Impact of Hospital Market Structure on Patient Volume, Length of Stay, and Cost of Care 1972–82." *Journal of Health Economics* 4: 333–56.

———. 1987. "Competition and the Cost of Hospital Care 1972–82." *Journal of the American Medical Association* 257: 3241–45.

———. 1988. "Competition, Regulation, and Hospital Costs 1982–1986." *Journal of the American Medical Association* 260: 2676–81.

Russell, L. 1989. *Medicare's New Hospital Payment System: Is It Working?* Washington, DC: Brookings Institution.

Schieber, G. J., and J. P. Poullier. 1990. "Overview of International Comparisons of Health Care Expenditures." In *Health Care Systems in Transition*, 9–15. Paris: Organization for Economic Cooperation and Development.

Schwartz, W., and D. Mendelson. 1991. "Hospital Cost Containment in the 1980s: Hard Lessons Learned and Prospects for the 1990s." *New England Journal of Medicine* 324: 1037–42.

Stokey, E., and R. Zeckhauser. 1978. *A Primer of Policy Analysis.* New York: W. W. Norton & Co.

Swint, J. M. 1990. *International Summit on the Economic Impact of Health Care Systems.* Houston: University of Texas Health Science Center, Health Policy Institute.

Torrance, G. W., M. H. Boyle, and S. P. Horwood. 1982. "Application of Multiattribute Utility Theory to Measure Social Preferences for Health States." *Operations Research* 30: 1043–69.

Warner, K. E., and B. R. Luce. 1982. *Cost-Benefit and Cost-Effectiveness Analysis in Health Care.* Ann Arbor: Health Administration Press.

Williams, A. H. 1974. "Need as a Demand Concept (with Special Reference to Health)." In *Economic Policies and Social Goals: Aspects of Public Choice*, edited by A. J. Culyer, 60–76. London: Martin Robertson.

———. 1990. "Ethics, Clinical Freedom and the Doctor's Role." In *Competition in Health Care: Reforming the NHS*, edited by A. J. Culyer, A. K. Maynard, and J. W. Posnett, 178–91. London: MacMillan Press.

Woolhandler, S., and D. Himmelstein. 1991. "The Deteriorating Administrative Efficiency of the U.S. Health Care System." *New England Journal of Medicine* 324: 1253–58.

Zwanziger, J., and G. Melnick. 1988. "The Effects of Hospital Competition and the Medicare PPS Program on Hospital Cost Behavior in California." *Journal of Health Economics* 7: 301–20.

Chapter 5

Efficiency: Evidence and an Application

This chapter examines the evidence on the efficiency of the U.S. medical care system and, in particular, the relationship between physician payment and efficiency. The chapter reviews both micro evidence, i.e., the average efficiency of physicians, hospitals, and insurers in comparison to the achievable minimum cost, and the macro evidence, i.e., the performance of the U.S. medical care system in comparison to other Western nations.

Evidence Relating to the Efficiency of Medical Care

Allocative efficiency

A basic conclusion of Chapter 3 was that medical care may have little to do with health compared to genetics, environment, and behavior. Thus, critics have long been concerned that modern developed countries allocate too many resources to the delivery of personal health services and too few to activities that would improve the physical and social environment (Fuchs 1974; McKeown 1990). This concern is at the core of the debate between medicine and public health. McKeown (1990, 85) summarizes the public health position as follows:

> What health services need in general is an adjustment in the distribution of interest and resource between prevention of disease, care of the sick who require investigation and treatment, and care of the sick who do not need active intervention. Such an adjustment must pay considerable attention to the major determinants of health: to food and the environment, which

will be mainly in the hands of specialists, and to personal behavior, which
should be the concern of every practicing doctor.

The great improvements in health over time have been primarily due
to public health measures that were enabled by economic development
and growth. Even in the case of medical breakthroughs in treatment
of deadly communicable diseases, delivery of these personal medical
services lagged behind the decline in disease (McKeown and Lowe 1974).
After reviewing historical data on medicine and health, McKeown and
Lowe conclude that specific medical preventive and therapeutic efforts
played a minor role in the reduction in mortality from the eighteenth century to the present. The most important factors were an improvement in
nutrition from the early eighteenth century and limitation in population
growth and improvement in hygiene from the late nineteenth century.
Evans and Stoddart (1990) have suggested that medical care spending
has risen to the point where it may actually cause a decline in the health
of the population because it takes resources from areas like education,
housing, and the environment that have a positive contribution to health
and applies them to medical services that have low, no, or even negative
impacts on health.

Despite the critics, modern medicine does provide many benefits
and is in great demand by people throughout the world. However,
there is concern that we spend too much on treatment and too little
on preventive services. For example, those aged 65 and over consumed
35 percent of the health care dollar in 1984 (Waldo and Lazenby 1984),
and the 5.9 percent of Medicare beneficiaries who died in 1978 accounted
for 28 percent of Medicare reimbursements, with 60 percent of that
expenditure coming in the last 30 days of life (Lubitz and Prihoda 1984).
This has raised questions about a possible misallocation of scarce medical
resources (Scitovsky 1988). However, the prognostic skills of physicians
still do not permit a determination of who among survivors would have
died but for the care they received (Webster and Berdes 1990). While the
spending pattern that favors treatment may seem irrational from a public
policy standpoint, it makes good sense from a consumer-sovereignty,
individual-choice perspective. One reason so little preventive health care
is consumed is because it is often not insured. Insurance is most desirable
for uncertain events that are costly when they occur. Preventive services
are generally not expensive and can be planned. Also, it is rational for
individuals to have a high demand for health services when they are
ill, even when the effect is uncertain, and a low demand for preventive
services when they are well.

When Oregon attempted to assign priorities to services and fund
them on a cost-effectiveness basis, the public rejected the ranking because

the proposed system ranked some effective services that could save lives but would benefit relatively *few* people, e.g., appendectomy, below services that could provide a small improvement in quality of life for *many* people, e.g., dental caps (Hadorn 1991). The rejection of the rational cost-effectiveness model is attributed to the "rule of rescue" (Jonsen 1986). People cannot stand by when a known person's life is threatened and something can be done about it. This is so even when the cost is enough that investing the same funds in preventive programs would save several unknown persons in the future.

Even so, as a nation, we may be overspending on personal health services to the neglect of areas that may have a greater effect on health. In 1990, national health expenditures were $666.2 billion, of which $585.3 billion (87.9 percent) was for personal health care, $19.3 billion (2.9 percent) was for government public health activities, and $12.4 billion (1.9 percent) was for research and development. The remaining expenditures were for program administration and the net cost of private insurance, $38.7 billion (5.8 percent) and construction $10.4 billion (1.6 percent) (Levit et al. 1991).[1]

The U.S. Department of Health and Human Services (1990) reports an allocation of $4.9 billion to preventive activities in 1987 and $5.2 billion in 1988. Recently, there has been a shift toward greater reimbursement and provision of preventive services. The continuing growth of health maintenance organizations, which typically provide a broad range of preventive care, is a major factor. HMOs now cover about 13 percent of the population, and payers continue to look to them to provide access to comprehensive care with cost control. Studies of effectiveness and cost-effectiveness (Eddy 1980) have been used in selecting preventive services to be covered by insurance (Preventive Services Task Force 1989). The Blue Cross and Blue Shield Association has issued guidelines for a lifetime schedule of medical tests to detect adult disease. Preventive services will be insured if subscribers choose to pay the additional cost of about $90 a year for a family or $36 for an individual (Pear 1991a). Medicare now covers selected preventive services such as Pap smears and is considering other preventive services for the elderly. Medicaid, in many states, has long provided preventive services such as screening, immunizations, and preventive dental care.

Even within treatment, there is concern about misallocation of resources toward technical procedures and away from services that improve patient understanding of their health problems and what they can do to ameliorate and possibly avoid them in the future. Due to the malpractice and reimbursement systems, physicians are induced to perform procedures such as surgery and diagnostic tests and spend less time in taking histories and providing health education or motivational counseling to patients (cognitive services). Extensive testing provides documentation to use in the case of a medical liability lawsuit. Tests and other procedures also provide much higher remuneration per unit of time compared to cognitive services (Hsaio et al. 1988a). This problem is exacerbated by physician ownership of diagnostic equipment and laboratories (Hillman et al. 1990). Given that most diseases have a strong behavioral component, one of the most important and potentially effective aspects of patient care is being neglected by concentrating on procedures as opposed to patient education and counseling.

The RAND Health Insurance Experiment

The RAND Health Insurance Experiment, referred to in Chapter 3, addressed the allocative efficiency of coinsurance in the context of the U.S. medical care financing and delivery system. The study examined the effect of copayments on utilization and expenditures for medical care services and the extent to which increases in utilization associated with "free" care affected health status. The basic finding was that free care, compared to higher copayment levels, resulted in a 50 percent increase in expenditure with no significant effect on the health status of the typical person. Those, however, who were sick or poor, or both, at the time of enrollment obtained significant health status benefits from increased utilization. Reducing the price to the "typical" consumer below the cost of production, results in consumption of services, the marginal value of which is below the marginal cost of production (with little or no effect on health). This is the basic condition of resource misallocation. It implies that resources would provide more benefit if allocated elsewhere.

By applying the consumer-sovereignty framework to the Health Insurance Experiment findings, Manning et al. (1987) estimated that out of the $200 billion the under-65 population of the United States spent on health care in 1984, a $37-billion to $60-billion welfare loss (the allocation of resources to procedures or services with no or minimal benefits) would have been incurred by moving from the 95 percent copayment plan with a $1,000 maximum out-of-pocket expenditure to the free plan. This is the estimated amount of overspending that would have occurred under the free plan given the low marginal value of the added medical care services that would have been consumed. The authors note that some strong assumptions required to obtain this estimate might not hold and might therefore lead to an overestimate of loss. However, this is probably more than offset by the fact that the estimate ignores the incentives to employ new technologies associated with more-generous insurance plans. New technology is often used in ways that produce low marginal benefits for patients relative to cost, thereby *adding* to welfare loss.

The above welfare loss estimate is based on the current structure of the U.S. medical care system with its mix of regulatory and competitive features. Therefore, the estimate does not represent a forecast of the effects of fundamental restructuring of the medical care delivery and financing system to approximate systems in Canada or Europe. While those systems provide first-dollar coverage they also include budget caps, volume controls, and stringent control over capital expenditure on health care technology and facilities. An important perspective on the U.S. system is gained by comparing our spending, utilization, coverage, and health outcomes with those of other democratic industrialized countries. Differences are often not clearly associated with policy, but they raise questions about the performance of our system and achievable targets.

Macro evidence

The OECD has provided comprehensive health status, health care utilization, health resource, and health care expenditure data on its 24 member countries. These are democratic countries that range from economic powers such as the United States, Germany, and Japan to smaller countries with more modest economic achievement such as Greece and Portugal. While there are some problems with data comparability across countries (Schieber and Poullier 1990), the differences between the United States and other major countries demand explanation and raise questions about the efficiency of the U.S. system.

Table 5.1 shows a comparison among seven of the major, industrialized, OECD member countries: Canada, France, Germany, Italy, Japan, the United Kingdom, and the United States. With 11.2 percent of its GDP directed to health care in 1987, the United States spent 2.6 percentage points more than the second-ranked country, Canada. The U.S. per capita health care expenditure was $2,051 in 1987, about 40 percent more than Canada and 2.7 times more than the seventh-ranked country, the United Kingdom. This large expenditure gap was apparently not offset by health outcome advantages for the United States, which had the highest infant mortality level of the seven countries and life expectancy figures that were lower than most of the other countries. Furthermore, the United States was the only country of the seven with a significant population lacking health insurance—over 35 million people.

In addition to concern about misallocating resources to services that provide low benefit relative to cost, there is concern that medical care services of given quality are not provided at minimum cost. While the least-cost production scale and methods are difficult to determine for medical services, several studies have produced evidence of inefficient production.

Table 5.1 Comparative Health Care System Data for Seven Industrialized Countries, 1987

Country	Health Care Expenditures as Percentage of GDP	Health Care Expenditures per Capita in U.S. $	Population Uninsured	Percentage of Population Eligible for Public Insurance for Hospital Care	Infant Mortality per 1,000 Live Births	Life Expectancy at Birth in Years	
						Male	Female
United States	11.2	2,051	35 million	43	10.0	71.5	78.3
Canada	8.6	1,483	nil	100	7.9	73.0	79.8
France	8.6	1,105	nil	99	7.6	72.0	78.7
West Germany	8.2	1,093	nil	92	8.3	71.8	80.3
Italy	6.9	841	nil	100	9.6	71.6	78.1
Japan	6.8	915	nil	100	5.0	75.6	81.4
United Kingdom	6.1	758	nil	100	9.1	71.9	77.6
Mean	8.1%	$1,178	—	91%	8.2	72.5	79.2

Source: Organization for Economic Cooperation and Development 1990.

Production efficiency

Contrary to planning models that use fixed ratios of physicians and hospital beds per 1,000 population, medical care services can be provided in many different ways with different combinations of personnel and capital, production unit sizes, and locations of service delivery. Production efficiency is achieved when production units are of optimal size and the mix of inputs is such that the marginal product per dollar of cost is equal across all inputs. Only then is the cost minimized for a given level of output of medical services.

Economists and other health services researchers have conducted numerous studies on production efficiency, concentrating on the size and personnel mix of physician practices, the bed size of community hospitals, inpatient versus outpatient service delivery, insurance administration, general administrative costs of health systems, and, to a lesser extent, on the economies of scale of a single technology, such as coronary bypass surgery (Ludbrook 1987).

Physician services

Reinhardt (1972) and Smith, Miller, and Golladay (1972) took different analytical approaches to the optimal use of physician aides, but arrived at the same general conclusion. Physicians could raise the productivity of their practices and lower the cost per office visit by employing more aides. Using 1967 nationwide data, Reinhardt found that solo physicians could employ four rather than two auxiliaries and increase the number of patient visits by 25 percent. Similarly, Smith, Miller, and Golladay (1972) found that adding one physician assistant to a primary care practice could increase productivity by 49 percent to 74 percent, from 147 visits per week to as many as 265 visits per week. Brown (1988) replicated the Reinhardt study with a larger 1976 national data set. He found that, on average, group physicians were 22 percent more productive than solo practitioners and that physicians were not using aides efficiently. Subsequent to Reinhardt's study, physicians had expanded the number of aides to the point where they overemployed clerical administrative aides and technicians. Physicians employed 1.54 aides per physician in 1970, and 2.25 in 1978. Only group practices were employing the efficient number of physician assistants, and that may be an important source of the efficiency advantage enjoyed by such groups. Since Brown's study, aide use has declined, to 1.74 aides per physician in 1985, suggesting that physician practices are becoming more efficient.

Studies on economies of scale in physician practice conclude that group practice is more efficient than the traditional solo practice of medicine. Lee (1990) has critically reviewed the literature on the economics of group practice, concluding that we know little about the economics of group practice and that existing conceptual models are inaccurate. Surveys show that most group practices are owned by physicians and that resource allocation is done cooperatively, not by individual physicians within the groups. Conceptual models have focused on the lack of incentives for productivity faced by individual physicians in groups. However, this lack is not likely to pose serious problems because decisions are made cooperatively. Empirical studies suffer from lack of control of factors that may affect efficiency in group medical practice. Most serious is the failure to capture accurately differences in the quality and mix of services actually provided.

There were 16,579 medical group practices in the United States in 1988. They comprised about 30 percent of all nonfederal physicians (American Medical Association 1990). Reinhardt (1975) found that physicians in group practices generated 5.0 percent more patient visits and 5.6 percent more patient billings than physicians in solo practices. A case study by Newhouse (1973) found slight economies of scale (the tendency for average cost to decline as scale of production increases) accrued to group practice, but the savings were offset by higher costs associated with x-inefficiency. Because of sharing arrangements, individual physicians were less likely to conserve resources.

Survivor analysis has been used to test for economies of scale in physician practice (Frech and Ginsburg 1974; Marder and Zuckerman 1985). In this type of analysis, the fastest-growing size of practice for a given period of time is judged most efficient. The number of group practices has been growing relative to solo practices during the period from 1965 to 1988, suggesting that group practice is more efficient than solo practice (American Medical Association 1990). Frech and Ginsburg (1974) found that during the period from 1965 to 1969, solo practice was very inefficient, with small groups of 3 to 7 physicians and large groups of more than 26 physicians being most efficient. Marder and Zuckerman (1985) also found large groups to be most efficient during the period from 1975 to 1980.

Medical practice and technology have changed dramatically during the last 25 years, permitting many more surgical and diagnostic services to be done in an outpatient setting. Capital required to provide more sophisticated outpatient services can be financed and efficiently utilized in group practice settings. In addition to production efficiencies of group practice, high practice start-up costs, greater competition in a period of growing supply and budget restraints, and national and state health policies that favor HMOs all point to continued growth in group medical practice.

Hospital services

Considerable research has been conducted on the degree to which community hospitals are subject to economies of scale. Similar to physician services, the methods of hospital cost function analysis have been somewhat crude because measures of input and output do not take account of the great complexity of hospital-based care (Berki 1972; Cowing, Holtmann, and Powers 1983). Nevertheless, Feldstein (1988) concludes that there are slight economies of scale, with the optimum-sized community hospital being between 200 and 300 beds. The cost curve is shallow, suggesting that there are not large savings associated with attaining the optimal size. While hospitals in the United States are increasing in size, the average number of beds per hospital is still less than 200 (National Center for Health Statistics 1991).

A more important issue for hospitals, and one that also raises the quality question, is the efficient size of a given service or department within the hospital (Grannenmann, Brown, and Pauly 1986). This may include everything from open heart surgery to the size of the laundry facility and has implications for whether a given hospital should provide the service or not. Luft, Bunker, and Enthoven (1979) have shown a positive relationship between volume of heart surgery and outcome. Thus, in cases where higher service volume results in improved outcomes, efficiency can be improved by producing services at a lower cost per unit and by achieving more positive outcomes. Whether determined by regulation or market competition, such specialized services should be regionalized.

Health plans

Another level of efficiency analysis has been conducted at the health plan system level, usually comparing HMOs with the more traditionally insured groups and their fee-for-service providers (Luft 1981). There are both allocative and production differences between plans, and it is very difficult to sort out the reason for cost differences. Do HMOs save because they allocate less to inpatient care and more to prevention, because they provide services at less cost, or because they simply restrict access to care, whether beneficial or not at the margin?

A thorough review of the literature by Luft (1981) and the RAND randomized experiment (Manning, Liebowitz, and Goldberg 1984) provide the best evidence. Luft concluded that HMOs provided care for 10 percent to 40 percent less than comparable fee-for-service systems, the quality was no worse on average, and that most of the savings were due to fewer hospital admissions. He could not tell whether admissions eliminated by HMOs were more or less discretionary than those retained.

Through randomization into one large well-established HMO, the RAND study supported Luft's conclusion. They found savings of 25 percent with no adverse health effects on the general population, although persons who were initially sick and poor at the beginning of the experiment did fare better under the free fee-for-service plan than in the HMO. Savings may be due to factors other than economies of scale and using the efficient mix of manpower. The change in financial incentives and better resource management may reduce x-inefficiency.

More recently, point-of-service HMOs, preferred provider organizations, self-insured plans with cost-control features, and other managed care fee-for-service plans have been added to the debate. HMOs and traditional plans have become more similar, and it is difficult to distinguish clearly the reason for any cost differences (Luft 1988). While many payers, especially business, question whether they accrue savings by enrolling beneficiaries in HMOs, there continues to be momentum for both public and private payers to shift to managed care plans.

Physician practice continues to move toward more efficient personnel mix and scale, the average size hospital is increasing, very expensive and difficult services are being regionalized, and the number of HMO systems and their enrollments are increasing. Nevertheless, the medical care system suffers from excess capacity, inappropriate and ineffective services, overproduction of procedure-oriented care, high administrative costs, and excess profits that accrue to providers. Policymakers continue to struggle to provide the right mix of regulation and market competition that will provide incentives and controls for the right type and amount of technological innovation, efficient production and allocation, and equity of access to medical care services. At a minimum, policy should provide incentives for providers to adopt efficient practices in delivering medical services and should reduce the conflicts between regulation- and competition-oriented means to achieve these objectives.

Summary

The evidence suggests that the mix of regulatory and market systems in the United States has not produced economic efficiency. Providers are not induced to choose efficient means of production, charge near the cost of services, and provide care that is most demanded or needed by consumers. Other democratic, developed countries appear to be more successful at controlling spending, insuring their populations, and achieving health outcomes as measured in the traditional ways. Whether they are truly more efficient is impossible to determine from aggregate data. Even so, attaining cost-control and access goals is an important social achievement.

Physician payment represents one aspect of the U.S. system that has contributed to inefficiency. The discussion that follows focuses on why the system leads to inefficiency, the types of inefficiency that are induced, the failure of the market to correct the problems, the government's regulatory solution for the Medicare program, and implications for the efficiency of the U.S. medical care system.

An Application: Physician Payment Reform

Our current system of physician payment is both unfair and a contributor to inefficiency. It is unfair because different amounts are paid to different physicians for the same procedure, depending on the physician's past record of charges. It is inefficient because, by paying physicians more per unit of time for procedures than for cognitive services, the system affects practice patterns and may result in overprovision of certain ineffective and costly procedures. Further, medical services in general, due primarily to third-party reimbursement, have been overvalued compared to other goods and services in the economy. A distorted price structure draws new physicians away from primary care and into procedure-oriented specialties such as surgery and radiology.

Evidence suggests that as many as 17 percent to 30 percent of frequently performed surgical and diagnostic services are inappropriate or not indicated and another 8 percent to 30 percent of surgeries and diagnostic procedures are of questionable value (Chassin, Kosecoff, and Park 1987). In addition, there is a shortage of primary care providers and an excess supply of surgeons and other procedure-oriented specialists. As discussed in Chapter 3, there is much concern about the effectiveness of services and the variations in practice patterns that are not associated with patient outcomes. Much care appears to be of questionable value, but incentives for the provision of that care are strong and direct under an insurance-financed, fee-for-service system.

Ineffective market and regulatory control of prices has resulted in payments that are higher than necessary to attract providers to the field of medicine. For example, the average gross earnings of a general practitioner in the United States were $174,000 in 1985, more than double the figure for Canada and three times the amount for the United Kingdom (Sandier 1990). Fuchs (1990) found that physician expenditures per capita were 1.72 times higher in the United States than in Canada in 1985. All of the difference was explained by higher prices. U.S. fees for procedures are three times as high as in Canada, with fees for evaluation and management services being 80 percent higher in the United States. Net incomes of physicians are only about one-third higher in the United

States than in Canada, despite the large fee differences. Fuchs speculates that this may be due to U.S. physicians' higher overhead expenses and lower work load. These payments support a system that thrives without minimizing the cost of producing a given quality of care.

Another side of our entrepreneurial system was recently revealed in the state of Florida, where it is common for physicians to invest in laboratories, diagnostic facilities, and physical therapy units. Facilities owned by physicians charged higher prices, provided more units of service per patient, and provided lower-quality services than comparable facilities not owned by physician investors (Pear 1991b). In a study of the frequency and cost of diagnostic imaging, Hillman et al. (1990) examined health insurance claims of 403,458 employees and dependents of large American corporations. They found that self-referring compared to radiologist-referring office-based physicians obtained imaging examinations four times more often and charged significantly more for examinations of the same complexity. This resulted in mean imaging charges up to 7.5 times higher for self-referring physicians. These findings point to the conclusion that the financing system can lead to inefficiency through overpayment, overutilization, and poor quality.

It has been apparent for some time that the customary, prevailing, and reasonable (CPR) system of paying physicians was unsound. Under this system, Medicare and many private insurers reimbursed the lower of the median charge by the physician for the service during the previous year (customary), the prevailing charge in the locality (75th percentile of customary charges), and the actual charge. However, the prevailing charge is limited according to an allowable percentage change from a base period. This represented a regulated market approach to pricing. The system itself affected the market, as many payers adopted the approach of paying according to what others were charging. The result was a greatly increased rate of inflation in physician prices (Frech and Ginsberg 1978). Prices could not be adjusted downward, even when justified. For example, many procedures are difficult and risky when first introduced and justify a relatively high price. As physicians obtain experience and develop improved methods of providing the service, it may become easier and less risky to perform, but prices are maintained at the higher level. Cataract surgery is a prime example, although the government eventually intervened to lower the price of this procedure under Medicare.

Given concern about the equity and efficiency associated with physician payment, William Hsaio, with assistance from the American Medical Association and numerous medical specialty groups developed the resource-based relative value scale. The attempt was to develop a set of administered prices that reflected relative market values of the cost of providing each service. Much of the cost is the "work" required to provide the service. Hsiao et al. (1988b) developed methods to measure work, including components of time, mental effort and judgment, technical skill, stress, and physical effort. Practice costs are also a key component. Congress mandated a new payment system in the Omnibus Budget Reconciliation Act of 1989. Changes include a new fee schedule based on the RBRVS model, charge limits, and volume performance standards (Physician Payment Review Commission 1991). The latter will act to adjust prices downward if physicians respond to lower payments by increasing volume of services. The new system was phased in for the Medicare program over a five-year period beginning in January of 1992. Aspects of the system will be adopted by other payers and therefore will be likely to have a major impact on the medical care sector.

Simulations performed on the first phase of the new RBRVS system predict major shifts in procedure payments and physician income by specialty and anticipate some behavioral responses by physicians to offset a potential loss in income. For example, payments for primary care services will increase by 30 percent while payments for major surgical procedures (e.g., coronary artery bypass and total hip replacement) will be reduced by 34 percent and 23 percent, respectively. Payments for diagnostic procedures will also decrease. Cardiovascular stress tests payment will be reduced by 39 percent, for example. Physicians who provide primarily evaluation and management services will see their Medicare payments increase by 29 percent (general practice), and 30 percent (family practice) by 1996 when the system is fully implemented. The average surgical specialty will suffer a decrease of 7 percent, with some subspecialties such as thoracic surgery experiencing reductions of as much as 14 percent (U.S. Department of Health and Human Services 1991).

While the system was initially designed to be budget-neutral, there is hope that it will lead to long-run savings for the Medicare program by reducing the overutilization of procedure-oriented care, improving the quality and appropriateness of care, and changing the distribution of physicians among specialties (Hsiao 1991). The Physician Payment Review Commission and HCFA will be closely monitoring and evaluating the effects of the new system. While some have argued for a demonstration and evaluation of the system on a regional basis, possibly comparing it to a negotiated-fee-structure model, it will be implemented for the entire country, as was the prospective payment system for hospitals.

Health services researchers will be challenged to evaluate the effects of the new system. How will it affect the production efficiency and allocative efficiency of the health care system? What are the short-term and long-term effects on the cost and patterns of medical care? How will the system affect the distribution of physicians and income between primary and specialty care and among the specialties? Finally, what effect will the system have on technological change, and what are the implications for both effectiveness and efficiency?

The major questions posed concerning the efficiency objective were: what combination of medical care goods and services will be produced with society's limited resources, how are they produced, and are we obtaining the maximum value in terms of consumer well-being? The corollary issues are: what fundamental mechanisms are available for making these decisions, and which approach will lead to the "best" performance for a given society?

There is considerable evidence that the United States does not achieve maximum value from the resources allocated to medical care services and may perform less well than many other developed countries. Indicators include evidence on variability in the use of services and the lack of effectiveness and appropriateness of many medical care procedures as documented in Chapter 3, substantial underinvestment in selected preventive services, including prenatal care, a focus on procedure-oriented care that is costly and may add little to health at the margin, high rates of spending, and a relatively poor showing on many indicators of the population's health compared to other countries. Additionally, numerous studies have documented that hospital, physician, and insurance services are not produced in the most efficient manner, and comparative data suggest that prices and associated incomes are higher than necessary to attract the required resources to health care. Evidence includes excess capacity, a lack of attention to the most efficient personnel mix, and a failure to take advantage of potential economies of scale.

Blame is placed on our peculiar mix of open-ended pluralistic financing, the lack of planning and effective regulation (i.e., relying on an imperfect private market and unregulated entrepreneurial providers), a federally subsidized medical technology industry, and a population with high and possibly unrealistic expectations about what medicine can contribute to health. As costs continue to increase, we struggle with a debate about the proper type and mix of government and market mechanisms to improve the performance of the medical care delivery system.

Should the United States move toward the proven macro approach practiced in Canada and western Europe of direct government and community control over spending, or to a restructured, managed market that regulates insurers and gives providers and consumers clear incentives for making efficient decisions at the micro level? Cost control achieved through the macro approach does not necessarily translate directly into efficiency, but micro incentives have yet to demonstrate the ability to control cost, making allocative efficiency unlikely. Only by studying alternative models that have been developed on a state, regional, or national basis and by measuring their effects on well-being and cost will we begin to discern more clearly the answer to the troubling question of how best to improve the efficiency of the U.S. medical care system.

Note

1. Spending for environmental activities (e.g., air and water pollution abatement, sanitation and sewage treatment, water supplies) is excluded from the national health accounts (Levit et al. 1991).

References

American Medical Association. 1990. *Medical Group Practice in the United States: Survey of Practice Characteristics*. Chicago: American Medical Association.

Berki, S. 1972. *Hospital Economics*. Lexington, MA: D. C. Heath and Company.

Brown, D. M. 1988. "Do Physicians Underutilize Aides?" *Journal of Human Resources* 23: 342–55.

Chassin, M. R., J. Kosecoff, and R. E. Park. 1987. "Does Inappropriate Use Explain Geographic Variations in the Use of Health Services? A Study of Three Procedures." *Journal of the American Medical Association* 258: 2533–37.

Cowing, T. G., A. G. Holtmann, and S. Powers. 1983. "Hospital Cost Analysis: A Survey and Evaluation of Recent Studies." In *Advances in Health Economics and Health Services, Volume 4*, edited by R. Scheffler and L. Rossiter. Greenwich, CN: JAI Press.

Eddy, D. 1980. *Screening for Cancer: Theory, Analysis, and Design*. Englewood Cliffs, NJ: Prentice-Hall.

Evans, R., and G. Stoddart. 1990. "Producing Health, Consuming Health Care." *Social Science and Medicine* 31: 1347–63.

Feldstein, P. J. 1988. *Health Care Economics*. New York: John Wiley & Sons.

Frech, H. E., and P. B. Ginsburg. 1974. "Optimal Scale in Medical Practice: A Survivor Analysis." *Journal of Business* 47 (1): 23–36.

———. 1978. *Public Insurance in Private Medical Markets*. Washington, DC: American Enterprise Institute.

Fuchs, V. 1974. *Who Shall Live?* New York: Basic Books.

———. 1990. "How Does Canada Do It? A Comparison of Physicians' Services in the United States and Canada." *New England Journal of Medicine* 323: 884–90.

Grannenmann, T. W., R. S. Brown, and M. V. Pauly. 1986. "Estimating Hospital Costs: A Multiple-Output Analysis." *Journal of Health Economics* 5: 107–27.

Hadorn, D. 1991. "Setting Health Care Priorities in Oregon: Cost-Effectiveness Meets the Rule of Rescue." *Journal of the American Medical Association* 265: 2218–25.

Hillman, B. J., C. A. Joseph, M. R. Mabry, J. H. Sunshine, S. D. Kennedy, and M. Noether. 1990. "Frequency and Costs of Diagnostic Imaging in Office

Practice: A Comparison of Self-Referring and Radiologist-Referring Physicians." *New England Journal of Medicine* 323: 1604–8.

Hsiao, W. C. 1991. "Changing Physician Payment: Will It Affect Total Cost?" In *The Future of Health Care: Public Concerns and Policy Trends.* Waltham, MA: Massachusetts Health Data Consortium, Inc., pp. 11–14.

Hsiao, W. C., P. Braun, D. Dunn, E. R. Becker, M. DeNicola, and T. R. Ketcham. 1988a. "Results and Policy Implications of the Resource-Based Relative Value Study." *New England Journal of Medicine* 319: 881–88.

Hsiao, W. C., P. Braun, D. Yntema, and E. R. Becker. 1988b. "Estimating Physicians' Work for a Resource-Based Relative Value Scale." *New England Journal of Medicine* 319: 835–41.

Jonsen, A. 1986. "Bentham in a Box: Technology Assessment and Health Care Allocation." *Law, Medicine and Health Care* 14: 172–74.

Lee, R. H. 1990. "The Economics of Group Practice: A Reassessment." In *Advances in Health Economics and Health Services Research,* edited by R. M. Scheffler and L. F. Rossiter, 111–29. London: JAI Press.

Levit, K. R., H. C. Lazenby, C. A. Cowan, and S. W. Letsch. 1991. "National Health Expenditures 1990." *Health Care Financing Review* 13 (1): 29–54.

Lubitz, J., and R. Prihoda. 1984. "The Use and Costs of Medicare Services in the Last 2 Years of Life." *Health Care Financing Review* 5 (3): 117–31.

Ludbrook, H. 1987. "Economic Appraisal and Planning Decisions for Health Technologies". In *Economic Appraisal of Health Technology in the European Community,* edited by M. F. Drummond, 120–35. Oxford: Oxford Medical Publications.

Luft, H. S. 1981. *Health Maintenance Organizations: Dimensions of Performance.* New York: Wiley Interscience.

———. 1988. "HMOs and the Quality of Care." *Inquiry* 25:147–56.

Luft, H. S., J. P. Bunker, and A. C. Enthoven. 1979. "Should Operations be Regionalized? The Empirical Relation between Surgical Volume and Mortality." *New England Journal of Medicine* 20: 1364–69.

Manning, W., A. Liebowitz, and G. A. Goldberg. 1984. "A Controlled Trial of the Effect of a Prepaid Group Practice on Use of Services." *New England Journal of Medicine* 310: 1505–10.

Manning, W., J. Newhouse, N. Duan, E. Keeler, A. Leibowitz, and S. Marquis. 1987. "Health Insurance and the Demand for Medical Care: Evidence from a Randomized Experiment." *American Economic Review* 77 (3): 251–77.

Marder, W. D., and S. Zuckerman. 1985. "Competition and Medical Groups: A Survivor Analysis." *Journal of Health Economics* 4 (2): 167–76.

McKeown, T. 1990. "Determinants of Health." In *The Nation's Health,* edited by P. R. Lee and C. L. Estes. Boston: Jones and Bartlett.

McKeown, T., and C. R. Lowe. 1974. *An Introduction to Social Medicine.* London: Blackwell Scientific Publications.

National Center for Health Statistics. 1991. *Health, United States, 1990.* DHHS Pub. No. PHS 91-1232. Washington, DC: U.S. Government Printing Office.

Newhouse, J. P. 1973. "The Economics of Group Practice." *Journal of Human Resources* 8 (1): 37–56.

Organization for Economic Cooperation and Development. 1990. Health Care Systems in Transition. SPS No. 7. Paris: Organization for Economic Cooperation and Development.

Pear, R. 1991a. "Insurer Offers Medical Screening as Part of Policy." *New York Times*, 19 June: 1.

————. 1991b. "Study Says Fees Are Often Higher when Doctor Has Stake in Clinic." *New York Times*, 9 August: A1.

Physician Payment Review Commission. 1991. *Annual Report to Congress*. Washington, DC: Physician Payment Review Commission.

Preventive Services Task Force. 1989. *Guide to Clinical Preventive Services: Report of U.S. Preventive Services Task Force*. Baltimore, MD: Williams and Wilkins.

Reinhardt, U. E. 1972. "A Production Function for Physician Services." *Review of Economics and Statistics* 54 (1): 55–66.

————. 1975. *Physician Productivity and the Demand for Health Manpower*. Cambridge, MA: Ballinger Publishing Company.

Sandier S. 1990. "Health Services Utilization and Physician Income Trends." In *Health Care Systems in Transition*. Paris: Organization for Economic Cooperation and Development. pp. 41–56.

Schieber, G. J., and J. P. Poullier. 1990. "Overview of International Comparisons of Health Care Expenditures." In *Health Care Systems in Transition*. Paris: Organization for Economic Cooperation and Development. pp. 9–15.

Scitovsky, A. A. 1988. "Medical Care in the Last Twelve Months of Life: The Relation between Age, Functional Status, and Medical Care Expenditures." *Milbank Quarterly* 66: 640–60.

Smith, K. R., M. Miller, and F. L. Golladay. 1972. "An Analysis of the Optimal Use of Inputs in the Production of Medical Services." *Journal of Human Resources* 7 (2): 208–55.

U.S. Department of Health and Human Services. 1990. *Prevention '89/90: Federal Programs and Progress*. Washington, DC: U.S. Government Printing Office.

————. 1991. "Rules and Regulations." *Federal Register* 56 (227): Monday, 25 November.

Waldo, D., and K. C. Lazenby. 1984. "Demographic Characteristics and Health Care Use and Expenditures by the Aged in the United States: 1977–1984." *Health Care Financing Review* 6 (1): 1–29.

Webster, J. R., and C. Berdes. 1990. "Ethics and Economic Realities: Goals and Strategies for Care toward the End of Life." *Archives of Internal Medicine* 150: 1795–97.

Chapter 6

Equity of Access:
Concepts and Methods

A question fundamental to considerations of *equity of access* to medical care is, does equity of access imply a *right* to medical care? This raises the corollary question, how might the equity goal of the U.S. medical care system be defined?

The policy debate on equity centers on the meaning and importance of assuring the population a right to medical care. This chapter (1) clarifies the equity objective of the U.S. medical care system by examining the ethical and empirical foundations of a right to medical care, and (2) describes the health services research methods used to examine the extent to which this objective has been achieved.

Health services research has played and continues to play an important role in the formulation and clarification of the equity objective. The research and recommendations of the early and influential Committee on the Costs of Medical Care (1927–32) anticipated and identified many of the problems and solutions that continue to be a focus of health policy and health services research considerations of equity (Anderson 1990; Committee on the Costs of Medical Care 1932; Roemer 1985).

The committee recommended that (1) medical services, both preventive and therapeutic, should be furnished largely by organized groups of physicians and other health professionals; (2) all basic public health services should be available to the entire population according to need; (3) the costs of medical care should be met on a group payment basis, through the use of insurance, taxation, or both; (4) the study, evaluation, and coordination of medical services should be important functions for every state and community, and the coordination of rural with urban services should receive special attention; and (5) the education of health professionals should be broadened to encompass attention to the social as well as technical aspects of medical practice.

The evolution and proliferation of an alphabet soup of medical care organizations (HMOs, PPOs, and IPAs, among others); the support of medical education, staff, and service delivery programs in areas of need; the development of local, state, and regional health planning efforts; and the growth of the role of private and public insurers in the decades following the CCMC study were, in fact, presaged by the recommendations of that blue-ribbon committee.

Surveys conducted by the CCMC also took an empirical look at the equity question in a way that continues to guide many contemporary studies of access. A central finding of CCMC population surveys, for example, was that lower-income groups suffered more illness but received less medical care than the well-to-do. The committee found that the cost burden fell disproportionately on those who were sickest, many of whom were not able to pay for care.

The growth of the private insurance industry from the first group health insurance plan (a precursor to Blue Cross) initiated in Dallas, Texas, in 1929 by Baylor University Hospital to cover public school teachers, and the growth of federally supported public coverage, culminating in the passage of Medicaid and Medicare legislation in the mid-1960s, mirror the evolution of a fundamental equity principle of third-party financing. *This principle is to reduce the burden of illness that any particular family or individual must bear, through sharing the financial responsibility or spreading the costs.*

The current status of public and private health insurance coverage in the United States calls into question the extent to which this principle of shared responsibility underlies the existing system of third-party payment. Employers increasingly seek to limit who would be included under the coverage they provide, and to reduce the share of premiums employers are obligated to pay. Insurers are seeking providers' involvement as decision makers or gatekeepers for the types of services to be rendered or approved for payment, as well as restricting the population they are willing to insure based on how risky and expensive they expect that population's care to be. Providers are affiliating with competitive, cost-effective practice organizations that put them in a better position to capture and maintain a share of the health care market. As a consequence, distinctions between their role as caring professionals serving their patients' physical needs and their role as fiduciary agents managing their own fiscal interests have become increasingly blurred. With diminished federal support for the Medicaid program during the past decade, the proportion of the poor population covered under Medicaid, the benefits and services provided, and the amounts paid to providers for patients covered under that program have declined. Medicare's prospective payment system gives rise to concerns that elderly patients are being discharged "quicker and sicker," and to a heightened awareness of the lack of an adequate and adequately financed system of long-term community and institutional care for this older population.

The gaps in the safety net of coverage resulting from these changes in the public and private health insurance markets have resulted in a substantial increase in the number of Americans who have no or inadequate health insurance. In addition, many hospitals and other providers that serve a disproportionate number of the aged, poor, and uninsured are facing serious financial problems due to a continuing increase in their burden of uncompensated or undercompensated care.

This emerging profile of the U.S. health care delivery system leads to serious questions about the equity or fairness of the system of care and financing. An important development in the policy debate on this issue is the promulgation of proposals for more universal or national health insurance. The issue and the debate are not new. The conceptual and empirical underpinnings for national health insurance were imbedded in the deliberations and recommendations of the Committee on the Costs of Medical Care. Policy consensus in the mid-1960s led to the social insurance–based Medicare program for the elderly and the welfare-based Medicaid program for the poor. The recognition of the gaps and limitations of private and public systems of financing in the late 1970s resulted in a proliferation of national health insurance proposals: in 1976 over 125 sponsors introduced 21 different such proposals in the U.S. Congress (Anderson 1990).

The discussion that follows seeks to clarify and define the goal of equity of access to medical care. The ethical and empirical aspects of equity will be examined in the context of the assumptions inherent in a right to medical care.

Conceptual Framework and Definitions

Concept of a right to medical care

Rights are like tickets for admission. They refer to "proper grounds for seeking or claiming something." "Proper grounds" may be based on relatively informal social rules (first come, first served) or more formal institutional roles (members can step to the head of the line). Implicit in these formal and informal guidelines are underlying moral or ethical considerations of what seems a fair way of resolving such claims when access to the means for satisfying them—like seats in a movie theater or tickets for a special exhibit—is limited. Further, these guidelines may remain relatively implicit moral tenets or be translated into explicit, formal laws or regulations—depending on the level of societal consensus regarding the seriousness of the claims and the best ways to address them (Dougherty 1988).

Rights and the benefits they provide are not without a price. Claims of rights generally imply a resulting monetary or nonmonetary burden of assuring that the desired benefits are distributed fairly. Rights may, for example, entail making demands on others either to forbear engaging in certain behaviors that might prevent benefits from being distributed (negative rights)—forbidding discrimination on the basis of sex or race, for example—or to compel certain actions to assure that benefits are provided (positive rights)—such as raising taxes or premiums to pay for them. Related to the issue of a right to medical care is the issue of fair distribution of the resulting benefits (claims) and burdens (costs) of care (Dougherty 1988).

The questions posed in clarifying the concept of equity are summarized in Figure 6.1: does equity of access imply a *right* to medical care, *where a right involves claims against others for medical care goods and services*, and what are the ethical principles for deciding what claims are fair, *where fair refers to a just allocation of benefits and burdens?*

Justice is the ethical principle central to the question of whether equity implies a *right* to medical care. Individuals and group claims of "entitlement" to care result in both benefits and burdens. Value judgments of who really is entitled and why are the crux of determining the fairness of the claims.

Equity or *distributive justice* is concerned with the fair allocation of benefits and burdens among those who are deserving of care and those who are in a position to pay for it—the two groups may or may not be the same. Micro-level decisions (by individual providers or institutions) that are guided by considerations of the principle of distributive justice include whether they will accept uninsured or Medicaid patients, and the types or intensity of services they are willing to render. Macro (societal or governmental) decisions include setting priorities regarding the benefits to be provided, the population to be covered, and the allocation of the costs of a universal health insurance plan.

Assumptions underlying the concept of a right to medical care invite a look both at the objectives of effectiveness, efficiency, and equity and at the balance and trade-offs among them. These assumptions include the following: (1) "right" refers to a right to *medical care*—not a right to *health*; (2) the resources for allocating medical care are finite; and (3) health policy should be concerned with the design of "just" mechanisms for allocating scarce medical care resources.

Figure 6.1 Concept of a Right to Medical Care

Major Issue

Does equity of access imply a *right to medical care,* where a *right* involves *claims* against others for medical care goods and services?

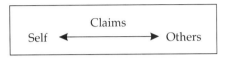

Corollary Issue

What are the ethical principles for deciding what claims are *fair,* where *fair* refers to a *just* allocation of benefits and burdens?

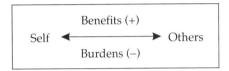

A right to health care or medical care is not the same as a right to health. A variety of personal factors (such as high-risk behaviors) or environmental correlates (such as persistent poverty or family violence) that lie outside the domain traditionally addressed by the medical care system may contribute to poor health. Evaluations of the *effectiveness of medical care* are therefore helpful in informing policymakers regarding the services for which it would be most prudent for rights (claims) to be granted. Commitments to improve *health* may, however, extend beyond societal assurances of access to medical care alone.

Recognition of the finitude of medical care resources raises the question of how best to allocate these resources to realize desired goals. The application of principles of allocative and production efficiency helps to assure the most *efficient* use of scarce medical care resources. The efficient operation of the medical care system also results in more resources being freed for other desired purposes (such as investments in public health or education).

At the heart of the concept of justice as applied to medical care is the issue of what criteria define a just system for allocating scarce medical care resources (Aday and Andersen 1981). The discussion that follows provides an ethical compass for directing empirical inquiries into this difficult normative question. The conceptual points of reference for such an inquiry are the divergent (and often contradictory) theoretical perspectives that define the concept of justice itself.

Theories of distributive justice (equity)

Different theories of justice emphasize different principles for a fair distribution of benefits and burdens as the foundation for defining the nature and limits of a right to medical care (Daniels 1985; Dougherty 1988). (See Table 6.1.)

Entitlement

Robert Nozick's entitlement theory emphasizes that fairness is rooted in the freedom to possess and use one's property and resources as one chooses (Nozick 1974). People are entitled to what they have as long as they acquire or transfer it through just means, that is, through their own labor or as a result of a gift, an inheritance, or a voluntary exchange with others. Further, the state should not interfere with or attempt to regulate these transactions. Instead, the "invisible hand" governing the free marketplace should be allowed to operate unhindered. The only appropriate intrusions would be to correct situations in which there is clear historical evidence that the property or resources some people possess were not acquired through just means. Such evidence is often difficult to assemble or document, however. Entitlement theory underlies market-based, pro-competitive approaches to health care policy. This perspective endorses policies that maximize consumer choice and satisfaction (preferences) in the medical care marketplace.

Egalitarian

From an *egalitarian* point of view, what is primary is the perspective that all individuals are of equal worth and should be treated equally. As Robert Veatch and others have pointed out, egalitarianism may focus on procedural or substantive equality—similarity in treatment or outcome, respectively (Veatch 1981). Procedural equality assures equal opportunity for *every* individual to obtain care, regardless of personal characteristics, such as age, gender, race, income, type of coverage, or whether one lives in the city or suburbs. Substantive equality emphasizes minimizing the health status differentials or variations between groups (such as black-white disparities in infant mortality). Considerations of positive rights to medical care from an egalitarian point of view focus on how to narrow or eliminate these disparities in health and medical care.

Table 6.1   Theories of Distributive Justice

Entitlement Theory

Major Theorist: Robert Nozick

Major Principles: *Entitlement*:
Individuals are entitled to what they possess, provided they acquire and transfer it through just means.

Libertarianism:
The state should not enforce these property rights and *not* interfere in redistributing it, i.e., let "the invisible hand" work.

Egalitarian Theory

Major Theorist: Robert Veatch

Major Principles: *Equal Worth*:
Principle of equality rests on the assumption of the equal intrinsic *worth* of all human beings.

Equal Opportunity:
Everyone has a claim to the health care needed to provide an opportunity for a level of health equal, as far as possible, to other persons' health.

Contractarian Theory

Major Theorist: John Rawls

Major Principles: *Greatest Equal Liberty*:
Every person should have an equal right to the most extensive system of equal basic liberties compatible with a similar system of liberty for all.

Fair Equality of Opportunity:
Persons with similar abilities and skills are to have equal access to offices and positions.

Difference Principle:
Social and economic institutions should be arranged to benefit maximally the *worst* off.

Needs-Based Theory

Major Theorist: Norman Daniels

Major Principles: *Normal Species Functioning*:
Meeting health care needs helps to maintain normal species functioning, and normal species functioning in turn has a major impact on an individual's share of the normal opportunity range.

Continued

Table 6.1   Continued

Fair Equality of Opportunity:
Society should be concerned with providing care that guarantees a fair equality of opportunity for normal functioning.

Utilitarian Theory

Major Theorists: David Hume
                   Jeremy Bentham
                   John Stuart Mill

Major Principles: *Utility*:
                   Promote the greatest good for the greatest number.

                   Teleological (Consequentialist):
                   Gauge the worth of actions by their consequences, i.e., the end justifies the means.

Contractarian

John Rawls's contractarian theory is based on an argument regarding what reasonable people would decide if they were asked to come together to derive a fair set of principles for distributing societal goods, operating under the hypothetical assumption that they could by chance be in *any* position in a society in which such principles would be applied (including the least advantaged socially or economically) (Rawls 1971). Rawls reasoned that such people would endorse the following principles, in order of importance: (1) maximize everyone's rights to liberties compatible with a similar system of liberty for everyone, (2) assure fair equality of opportunity for people with similar abilities and skills, and (3) make sure that those who are worst off benefit. The first two principles have a strong egalitarian orientation, and the third emphasizes that if any group "counts" more than another, it is those who are worst off, financially or otherwise. This perspective focuses on assuring the rights of those least able to buy care or be cured.

Needs-based

Norman Daniels's needs-based theory of justice points out that medical care is necessary to address minimal human needs for "normal species functioning" (Daniels 1985). Rights to medical care are justified in terms of their role in assuring that there is a fair equality of opportunity for living a normal life, which relates to a fundamental tenet of Rawls's contractarian theory as well. This perspective prompts consideration of what such needs might be, and the basic, decent minimum set of services that should be provided to meet them. Daniels suggests the following for consideration: adequate nutrition and shelter; sanitary, safe, unpolluted living and working conditions; exercise, rest, and features of a healthy lifestyle; preventive, curative, and rehabilitative personal medical services; and nonmedical personal (and social) support services.

Utilitarian

Utilitarian theory has its origins in the writings of David Hume, Jeremy Bentham, and John Stuart Mill (Dougherty 1988). It is principally consequentialist or ends-oriented. The value of any decision or action is judged by its consequences: "the end justifies the means." The principal goal is to maximize utility—to promote the greatest good for the greatest number. Cost-benefit- and cost-effectiveness-oriented decision making and market-oriented policies are rooted in the utilitarian perspective. Utilitarians advocate medical care rights that assure access to those services for which the measured benefits (in terms of health, well-being, or productivity, for example) would be maximized relative to what it costs to provide them (Culyer 1992).

Summary

Based on the varying concepts of distributive justice and associated rights reviewed above, the answer to the first question posed in this chapter, does equity of access imply a *right* to medical care, is that such a right is either an implicit or an explicit component of the equity objective. Many of the criteria used in evaluating the fairness of the current system of medical care delivery and financing in the United States derive from these theoretical perspectives on justice.

Ethical and empirical foundations of the goal of equity of access to medical care

The major goals for equity of access to medical care include (1) maximizing consumer choice; (2) not discriminating on the basis of such factors as age, sex, race, or ability to pay; (3) assuring some minimum standards for everyone; (4) making sure those who need care get it; and (5) providing high-quality care at an affordable cost. These commonly applied norms of distributional fairness parallel ethical principles derived from the major theoretical perspectives on justice: (1) freedom of choice, (2) similar treatment, (3) decent, basic minimum, (4) need, and (5) cost-effectiveness (Aday and Andersen 1981; Outka 1975). Conflicts over the interpretation or operating definitions of these norms and the relative importance assigned to each fuel debates regarding how to design equitable health care programs and policies.

Based on these varying criteria, the response to this chapter's second question, how might the equity goal of the U.S. medical care system be defined, is, "*to provide* the freedom and equality of opportunity *to obtain* adequate and effective medical care." This goal attempts to incorporate and balance the variety of competing criteria for evaluating the fairness of the medical care system, and reflects the implicit or explicit elements of a right to medical care embodied in alternative theories of distributive justice.

Table 6.2 summarizes the ethical and empirical foundations for the objective. This goal focuses on the manner and extent to which care is both provided (made available) and obtained (used). How care is provided is theoretically essential to and largely determinant of how care is used. Empirically, the goal recognizes the effect of potential access barriers (a lack of obstetrics providers in rural or inner-city areas) on realized access (the proportion of women who seek prenatal care) for a given population (high-risk mothers). Providers and consumers of care assume benefits and burdens. The intent of the objective is that ultimately people *obtain adequate and effective medical care*. The effectiveness and efficiency criteria described in previous chapters are essential and interrelated considerations in determining what is adequate and effective.

The equity objective has traditionally been examined empirically in the context of access. Access refers to the potential and actual entry of a given population group to the medical care system. The probability of entry is influenced by the structure of the delivery system itself (the availability, organization, and financing of services) and the nature of the wants, resources, and needs of potential consumers. The realization of the objective of entry is reflected in the population's objective rates of utilization, as well as in patients' subjective evaluations of the care they ultimately obtain (Aday, Andersen, and Fleming 1980).

The discussion that follows highlights key indicators of potential or realized access that can be used as empirical measures of equity. The next chapter presents research evidence regarding how well the system is performing in terms of these criteria.

Freedom of choice

Concept. The freedom-of-choice principle conforms most closely to Nozick's entitlement concept of justice. This principle emphasizes the importance of maximizing satisfaction of individual tastes and preferences in determining who gets what types of care. Proponents of this approach endorse the operation of the market-based forces of supply and demand for the allocation of medical care.

Table 6.2   Ethical and Empirical Foundations of the Goal of Equity of Access to Medical Care

Goal of Equity of Access to Medical Care	Criteria of Equity	Dimensions of Access	Indicators of Equity of Access
To Provide		*Potential Access*	
The freedom and	Freedom of choice	Characteristics of the delivery system	
		—Availability	Distribution of providers
		—Organization	Types of facilities
		—Financing	Sources of payment
Equality of opportunity	Similar treatment	Characteristics of the population	
		—Predisposing (age, sex, race, education)	
		—Enabling (income, regular source, insurance)	Regular source of care Insurance coverage
		—Need (perceived, evaluated)	
To Obtain		*Actual Access*	
Adequate and	Decent basic minimum	Type of utilization	Use of selected services
Effective	Need	Purpose of utilization	Use of services relative to need
	Cost-effect- iveness		
		Satisfaction	
		—General	Public opinion
		—Visit-specific	Patient opinion
Medical care			

Indicators. Empirical indicators of access, based on the freedom-of-choice norm, are the distribution and availability of medical care resources to consumers. For example, personnel- (e.g., primary care physicians or specialists) and facility- (e.g., hospitals or hospital beds) to-population ratios and related inventories of medical personnel or providers (e.g., HMOs, PPOs) in a given target (or market) area are indicators of the basic supply of providers and delivery sites available to consumers.

Lists of preferred providers affiliated with employer-sponsored health insurance plans also effectively define the range of enrollees' choices for a regular source of medical care. Other indicators of the extent to which patients' decisions may be constrained include data on the hours of clinic operation and provider availability at night, on weekends, or in emergencies; the average distance to the nearest medical facility and the modes of transportation for getting there; and the average time it takes to get an appointment to be seen, as well as the waiting time to see a physician or other provider once at the site.

Characteristics of the system of financing in an area—such as the generosity of a state's Medicaid program, the type and scope of benefits provided by major employers, and the local public or private arrangements for people who have no third-party coverage—also dictate the options consumers can realistically afford. Substantial cost-sharing provisions or uncovered medical expenses can also result in decisions to forgo goals or sacrifice personal resources intended for other uses—such as an elderly woman having to use her and her husband's life savings (or "spend down"), until he can qualify for nursing home coverage under Medicaid.

Similar treatment

Concept. The principle of similar treatment is a defining tenet of the egalitarian concept of justice. Fein (1972) refers to distributive justice derived on this basis as "vertical equity, that is, those who have the least status and power in a society should be treated no worse than the rich and powerful. This principle emphasizes that age, sex, race, income, or whether a person is covered by Medicaid, private insurance, or no insurance should not dictate that people with similar needs enter different doors (e.g., private physicians' offices versus hospital emergency rooms) or be treated differently (in terms of the type or intensity of services provided) by the medical care system.

Indicators. The similar treatment norm attempts to evaluate intergroup differences that may indicate inequalities in access to medical care. The convenience and characteristics of the places people go for medical care provide data on whether there is differential "treatment" of individuals in these different settings. Nonmedically motivated transfers of patients ("dumping"), principally as a function of fiscal rather than physical diagnostics ("wallet biopsies"), are indicative of inequity, applying the similar-treatment norm. Certain institutions or providers assuming a disproportionate burden of uncompensated care for the medically indigent population calls into question whether they are assuming more than their fair share from an egalitarian point of view.

Decent, basic minimum

Concept. Some critics have argued that a fairer alternative to the unfettered operation of the medical care marketplace is the assurance of some basic minimum of care for everyone, with market forces being allowed to operate in allocating services beyond this minimum. In contrast to strict egalitarianism, consumers with more resources would have the freedom and opportunity to purchase medical care above the minimum (Blumstein and Zubkoff 1979; Fein 1972; Fried 1976).

A major problem of the decent, basic minimum set of services is how to decide what and how much should be included (Agich and Begley 1985). Norman Daniels's formulation of requirements to maximize human functioning implies a broad array of medical care and related public health and social services. Considerations of the continuum of caring required to deal with health care problems would similarly include primary care, acute medical care, and long-term care services, at a minimum. Though a variety of norms may come into play in efforts to define a decent, basic minimum set of services, this framework provides a basis for assessing that to which individuals might have a right at different stages of care seeking.

Indicators. The decent, basic minimum standard can be measured through the type and comprehensiveness of services included in a given health benefit package. A core set of federally mandated benefits are covered under the Medicaid program and HMO legislation, but the states and plans, respectively, decide what optional services to offer (such as prescribed drugs, dental care, personal care, or podiatrist or other professional services, among others). Oregon's efforts to assign priorities to the various services covered under the Medicaid program in that state have raised a considerable hue and cry about fairness, which led in 1992 to the Health Care Financing Administration declining to grant a waiver enabling the Oregon Medicaid program to enact these provisions (Eddy 1991; Hadorn 1991). An assumption underlying the diagnosis-related group method of reimbursing hospital services under Medicare is that an appropriate bundle of services for addressing patients' needs can be specified. Critics of these payment methods have, however, argued that elderly Medicare patients are being discharged "quicker and sicker," without adequate provisions for long-term care (Kosecoff et al. 1990; Sager et al. 1989; Wood and Estes 1990).

Need

Concept. Rawls's contractarian theory of social justice, as well as Daniels's needs-based theory of equity, lend support to a primary focus on meeting basic *needs* as the criterion for the allocation of medical care. Assessing who "needs" care may be both difficult and expensive (Braybrooke 1987). Economic theory argues that expressed demand is the most rational basis for allocating scarce medical care resources. Needs may, in fact, be quite subjective and ungovernable, unless constrained by some sense that people are willing to pay to have their tastes and preferences satisfied. Further, societal or professional consensus may be required to determine which needs to meet when resources are limited.

Indicators. Indicators of equity from the perspective of need attempt to assess the magnitude of met or unmet medical need in a population. Sometimes survey respondents are asked questions to obtain their subjective perceptions of the extent to which their needs have been met: "During the past year, did you or a family member need to see a doctor but not see one for some reason? If so, why?" Other indicators summarize respondents' objective reports of the number of physician visits relative to the number of disability days they experienced in the year (use-disability ratio) or compare the number of people who actually contacted a physician for a set of symptoms with the number of people that a panel of physicians thought should have seen them for those symptoms (symptoms-response ratio) to assess the extent to which required services were actually obtained (Aday, Andersen, and Fleming 1980).

The fairness of the medical care system in the light of this criterion is also mirrored in ratios that compare realized access rates between groups—such as the simple ratio of the percentage of people with chronic illness who have been to a doctor in the past year among the poor and the percentage of such people among the nonpoor; the odds ratio (or likelihood) of having sought care during the first trimester of pregnancy for women on Medicaid compared to those with private coverage; and the percentage of deaths due to untreated hypertension among African Americans compared to the percentage among whites.

Cost-effectiveness

Concept. Based on the utilitarian theory of judging the rightness or wrongness of actions by the balance of benefits and burdens produced, cost-effectiveness and associated cost-benefit analyses have become an increasing focus in weighing the types of programs that should be funded and the categories of services to be covered under public or private insurance schemes. (The methods and measures used in cost-benefit and cost-effectiveness analysis were discussed in Chapter 4.) However, insurers may choose not to cover the most cost-effective services because of competing societal values or professional norms. Rosenblatt (1989), for example, describes the "perinatal paradox" entailed in policies that insure high-risk newborns have near-universal access to high-cost, life-saving neonatal intensive care technologies, but make no comparable assurance of access to adequate prenatal care. Prenatal services have been demonstrated to be highly cost-effective interventions to prevent adverse birth outcomes in the first place. The controversy over efforts to determine the core set of procedures and services to be covered under Medicaid in the state of Oregon has similarly pointed to a tendency on the part of both policymakers and the public to assign greater importance to identifiable individuals or lives, rather than the statistical aggregate numbers of lives saved, in evaluating policy options (Hadorn 1991).

An individual may be judged to need a certain procedure, but the costs of providing that procedure are high and the likely long-term benefits questionable in terms of improved quality or increased quantity of life. The difficulties and dilemmas of balancing need and cost-effectiveness norms have surfaced most directly in debates in Oregon regarding the criteria used in deciding what procedures and services should be covered under the Medicaid program in that state (Hadorn 1991). The initial cost-benefit calculus regarding what to include seemed to favor minor, less-costly treatments over costly lifesaving ones. In response to ethical criticisms, revisions were made that excluded cost per se and attempted to strike a balance between *need* and *effectiveness* criteria. Priority was assigned to those procedures that were estimated, in the aggregate, to yield the greatest probable health benefit, with cost being a secondary consideration. Attendant consideration was given to clinical guidelines to clarify the indications (or types of patients) for which specified services may be *most* necessary.

Indicators. A major focus of the Institute of Medicine report on *Access to Health Care in America* is the development of indicators of utilization relative to needs for which medical care can make a difference (visits for prenatal care, childhood immunizations, early cancer screening, and preventable hospitalizations, among others) (Institute of Medicine 1993). The findings from major health services research efforts, such as the RAND Health Insurance Experiment, the Medical Outcomes Study, and the AHCPR-sponsored medical-effectiveness and Patient Outcomes Research Team studies can provide an informed basis for identifying the most effective and efficient services for inclusion in a decent, basic minimum (and a maximum) of covered services (Agency for Health Care Policy and Research 1991; Lohr et al. 1986; Stewart et al. 1989).

Patient satisfaction is an indicator of realized access and the "good" that the client perceived resulted from care. People may be asked about their satisfaction with the medical care system in general, with their usual source of care, or with the care they received on their last visit. A number of satisfaction questions and scales have been developed for this purpose (Aday, Andersen, and Fleming 1980; Blendon and Taylor 1989; Hulka et al. 1975; Ware and Snyder 1975). Also, estimates of patients' perceptions of benefits from various treatment options are obtained by asking them about what trade-offs they would be willing to make, based on the probable outcomes of different options, e.g., five or more additional years of life requiring the use of aids for bowel and bladder function versus an uncertain prognosis involving the use of experimental drug therapy (Torrance 1986).

Summary

Implicitly or explicitly, the U.S. health care system goal of equity of access to medical care, as articulated here, assumes a commitment to assuring a limited right to medical care. The definition of the right implied in this objective is *to provide the freedom and equality of opportunity to obtain adequate and effective medical care.* This objective entails obligations and benefits for both the providers (or payers) *and* the consumers of medical care. The bottom line, however, is the universal provision of *adequate* and *effective* medical care.

Opinions will differ with respect to which components of this objective to emphasize, how to measure and implement it, and how well the current system, as well as proposals for change, might accomplish the objective. Health services research can assist in clarifying and informing the debate over these issues.

Key Methods of Assessing Equity of Access to Medical Care

Study designs

Three major types of health services research can help define and clarify the objective of equity, and how well programs and policies have succeeded in addressing it. These include descriptive, analytic, and evaluative health services research (Aday 1989).

Descriptive research focuses on profiling the access characteristics of the system. A variety of data sources provide basic information on the U.S. medical care system. Health services researchers use these sources in developing indicators of the main parameters and performance of the system with respect to equity of access. (See Table 6.2 and Appendix 7.1.)

Analytic research is directed toward understanding the relationship of system and population characteristics to achieving the outcome of the population's obtaining *adequate* and *effective* medical care. These studies are useful, for example, in illuminating the impact of policy-relevant variables, such as the type and extent of insurance coverage, on the use of services.

The framework Aday and Andersen developed for the study of access has guided a great deal of analytic research on equity. Integral to that framework is the value judgment that the system would be deemed fair or equitable if need-based criteria, rather than resources (such as insurance coverage or income), were the main determinants of whether or not and how much care is sought (Aday and Andersen 1981).

A particular challenge for health services researchers with respect to future analytic research on the equity objective defined here is identifying the types of medical care services that can eliminate or ameliorate need. Access to medical care for a problem that medical care cannot address poses the question of what *does* make a difference in preventing or remedying health problems. Analytic research on the correlates and consequences of health and human functioning can provide answers to questions regarding whether investments in medical care or in other systems or services are the most relevant bases for allocating scarce societal resources (Kaplan and Anderson 1988).

Evaluative research assesses how well programs and services that have been developed and implemented, based on previous descriptive and analytic research, have done in accomplishing equity of access. Evaluative studies rely primarily on quasi-experimental designs to determine program or policy outcomes. This research is particularly useful in informing policymakers regarding what programs or services work best and why. The RAND Health Insurance Experiment, for example, is an important social experiment that has made substantial methodological and substantive contributions to illuminating the effect of different health insurance alternatives on medical care utilization, cost, and outcomes. The findings from this study have provided a foundation for thinking about the future design of public and private systems of financing care.

Data sources

The primary focus of studies of access could be the medical care system as a whole, particular institutions within it, or the populations to be served by the system or facilities. Further, access studies could be carried out at the national, regional, state, or local (county or community) level. Such studies may entail collecting new (primary) data, as well as making use of data collected for other purposes (secondary data). Table 6.3 outlines the major types of primary and secondary data for assessing access at the system, institutional, and population level (Aday 1989; Aday, Sellers, and Andersen 1981).

Access descriptors at the *system* level focus on the availability, organization, and financing of services as aggregate, structural properties (Chitty and Schatz 1988; Kralovec and Andes 1988; National Center for Health Statistics 1989; Singer, Meyerhoff, and Schiffman 1985). Secondary data sources are most often used for this type of analysis. The Bureau of Health Professions, within the Health Resources and Services Administration, has, for example, compiled a computerized area resource file that has an array of health and health care data by county or metropolitan statistical area. The American Medical Association and the American Hospital Association, as well as other provider groups, routinely publish directories, and in some instances, have computerized data available on the characteristics and distribution of medical personnel. The National Center for Health Statistics collects data on the characteristics and utilization of hospitals, nursing homes, and outpatient medical care practices. The Health Care Financing Administration and the Health Insurance Association of America also periodically publish information on the amount and distribution of expenditures by the major public (Medicare and Medicaid) and private third-party payers. These data sources are particularly useful for describing the delivery system at the national, and to some extent, the state level.

Public health departments or private providers (such as national HMO firms considering entering a market) may want either more-current or more-detailed information on the types of services being provided or the profile of clients seen by facilities in a given area than is available from existing sources. In this case, the interested agencies or organizations

Table 6.3   Key Data Sources for Assessing Equity of Access to Medical Care

	Data Sources	
Study Universe	*Primary*	*Secondary*
System	Market area inventory	Area resource files
Institutions	Patient surveys	Patient records
Population	Population surveys	Census and other studies

Sources: Aday 1989; Aday, Sellers, and Andersen 1981.

could collect primary data, based on interviews with key community informants, telephone requests to providers for brochures describing their services, or full-fledged surveys of providers to gather data on the programs and services being offered and who is being served.

Secondary data used most often by *institutions* for assessing access to the facility include patient, financial, or other institutional records. Patient origin studies use patient address and zip code information to determine the areas from which most patients are drawn. If readily available in computerized files, patient record data could also serve as the basis for generating profiles of the demographic composition (age, sex, race) or the major presenting complaints of patients seen at the facility. Financial records also provide an indication of the level of uncompensated or undercompensated care the facility provides, and for what types of patients and services. Other institutional sources (such as clinic log books or emergency room referral records) are used in conducting studies of the magnitude and profile of unscheduled walk-in visits, and nonmedically motivated transfers within an institution.

Patient surveys are the major sources of primary data for evaluating access at the institutional level. Patient surveys tap individuals' *subjective* perceptions of their experiences at a given facility (how long they had to wait to be seen), which may or may not agree with more *objective* institutional records or data sources (average clinic waiting time estimates, for example). These subjective perceptions may, however, be more reflective of the extent to which people actually are satisfied and loyal users of a facility than would objective, records-based indicators.

Population-based studies of access include individuals who *may not* use a given delivery system or institution, as well as those who do. Surveys are particularly useful in measuring the attitudes or barriers that preclude targeted individuals or subgroups from seeking care. A number of large-scale, national surveys have examined access and trends over time for the U.S. population as a whole. These include the University of Chicago Center for Health Administration Studies series of utilization and access studies, the Robert Wood Johnson Foundation–Lou Harris surveys, the Agency for Health Care Policy and Research National Medical Care Expenditure surveys, and the continuing National Center for Health Statistics Health Interview Surveys, among others. Such surveys are, however, complex and expensive to conduct. State or local agencies may lack the resources and expertise for conducting such studies (Aday 1989).

Census or vital statistics data, and synthetic estimates, based on national sources, are some of the major types of secondary data used in profiling the actual or probable access of a population at the state or local level. Synthetic estimation procedures make use of data gathered at the national level (on utilization rates for certain age-sex-race groups) to impute what the estimates are likely to be at the state or local level (given the age-sex-race composition of the state or community) (Cohen 1980; DiGaetano et al. 1980; National Center for Health Statistics 1977).

The major question with which this chapter began was, does equity of access imply a *right* to medical care? The answer provided is that such a right is either an implicit or an explicit component of the equity objective. Whether or not rights to medical care evolve into legal entitlements depends on the outcomes of policy debates on the fairness of the claims.

The corollary question addressed in this chapter is, how might the equity goal of the U.S. medical care system be defined? The answer provided, based on a review of the conceptual and methodological contributions of health services research to studying equity, and in an attempt to integrate and focus competing views of fairness, is, "to provide the freedom and equality of opportunity to obtain adequate and effective medical care."

The particular challenges for health services researchers in terms of future descriptive, analytic, and evaluative research surrounding this objective are as follows:

— *Descriptive:* Identify or develop indicators of medical care use relative to needs for which medical care can make a difference.

— *Analytic:* Focus explanatory research on examining the effect of the organization and financing of medical care on patient outcomes.

— *Evaluative:* Evaluate existing or innovative models of care delivery and coverage with respect to their performance in providing adequate and effective care.

Chapter 7 reviews the empirical evidence on the extent to which the goal of equity of access to medical care in the United States has been achieved.

References

Aday, L. 1989. *Designing and Conducting Health Surveys: A Comprehensive Guide.* San Francisco: Jossey-Bass.

Aday, L., and R. Andersen. 1981. "Equity of Access to Medical Care: A Conceptual and Empirical Overview." *Medical Care* 19 (supp.): 4–27.

Aday, L., R. Andersen, and G. Fleming. 1980. *Health Care in the U.S.: Equitable for Whom?* Beverly Hills: Sage Publications.

Aday, L., C. Sellers, and R. Andersen. 1981. "Potentials of Local Health Surveys: A State-of-the-Art Summary." *American Journal of Public Health* 71: 835–40.

Agency for Health Care Policy and Research. 1991. *Report to Congress: Progress of Research on Outcomes of Health Care Services and Procedures.* AHCPR Pub. No. 91-0004. Rockville, MD: Agency for Health Care Policy and Research.

Agich, G., and C. Begley. 1985. "Some Problems with Pro-competition Reforms." *Social Science and Medicine* 21: 623–30.

Anderson, O. W. 1990. *Health Services as a Growth Enterprise in the United States since 1875,* 2d ed. Ann Arbor: Health Administration Press.

Blendon, R., and H. Taylor. 1989. "Views on Health Care: Public Opinion in Three Nations." *Health Affairs* 8 (March): 149–57.

Blumstein, J., and M. Zubkoff. 1979. "Public Choice in Health: Problems, Politics and Perspectives on Formulating National Health Policy." *Journal of Health Politics, Policy and Law* 4: 382–413.

Braybrooke, D. 1987. *Meeting Needs.* Princeton: Princeton University Press.

Chitty, M., and N. Schatz. 1988. *Federal Information Sources in Health and Medicine: A Selected Annotated Bibliography.* Westport, CT: Greenwood Press.

Cohen, S. 1980. "A Comparative Study of Synthetic Estimation Strategies with Applications to Data from the National Health Care Expenditures Study." In *Proceedings of the American Statistical Association, Section on Survey Research Methods.* Washington, DC: American Statistical Association, pp. 595–600.

Committee on the Costs of Medical Care. 1932. *Medical Care for the American People: The Final Report of the Committee.* Chicago: University of Chicago Press.

Culyer, A. J. 1992. "The Morality of Efficiency in Health Care—Some Uncomfortable Implications." *Health Economics* 1: 7–18.

Daniels, N. 1985. *Just Health Care.* Cambridge: Cambridge University Press.

DiGaetano, R., J. Waksberg, E. MacKenzie, and R. Yaffe. 1980. "Synthetic Estimates for Local Areas from the Health Interview Survey." In *Proceedings of the American Statistical Association, Section on Survey Research Methods.* Washington, DC: American Statistical Association, pp. 46–55.

Dougherty, C. 1988. *American Health Care: Realities, Rights, and Reforms.* New York: Oxford University Press.

Eddy, D. 1991. "Clinical Decision Making: From Theory to Practice—What's Going On in Oregon?" *Journal of the American Medical Association* 266: 417–20.

Fein, R. 1972. "On Achieving Access and Equity in Health Care." *Milbank Memorial Fund Quarterly/Health and Society* 50: 157–90.

Fried, C. 1976. "Equality and Rights in Medical Care." *Hastings Center Report* 6 (February): 29–34.

Hadorn, D. 1991. "Setting Health Care Priorities in Oregon: Cost-Effectiveness Meets the Rule of Rescue." *Journal of the American Medical Association* 265: 2218–25.

Hulka, B., L. Kupper, M. Daly, J. Cassel, and F. Schoen. 1975. "Correlates of Satisfaction and Dissatisfaction with Medical Care: A Community Perspective." *Medical Care* 13: 648–58.

Institute of Medicine. 1993. *Access to Health Care in America.* Washington, DC: National Academy Press.

Kaplan, R., and J. Anderson. 1988. "A General Health Policy Model: Update and Applications." *Health Services Research* 23: 203–35.

Kosecoff, J., K. Kahn, W. Rogers, E. Reinisch, M. Sherwood, L. Rubenstein, D. Draper, C. Roth, C. Chew, and R. Brook. 1990. "Prospective Payment System and Impairment at Discharge: The 'Quicker and Sicker' Story Revisited." *Journal of the American Medical Association* 264: 1980–83.

Kralovec, P., and S. Andes. 1988. *Inventory of U.S. Health Care Data Bases.* DHHS Pub. No. HRSA HRS-P-OD 88-2. Washington, DC: U.S. Government Printing Office.

Lohr, K., R. Brook, C. Kamberg, G. Goldberg, A. Leibowitz, J. Kessey, D. Reboussin, and J. Newhouse. 1986. "Use of Medical Care in the RAND Health Insurance Experiment: Diagnosis and Service-Specific Analyses in a Randomized Controlled Trial." *Medical Care* 24 (supp.): S1–87.

National Center for Health Statistics. 1977. *Synthetic Estimation of State Health Characteristics Based on the Health Interview Survey.* DHEW Pub. No. PHS 78-1349. Washington, DC: U.S. Government Printing Office.

———. 1989. *Data Systems of the National Center for Health Statistics.* DHHS Pub. No. PHS 89-1325. Washington, DC: U.S. Government Printing Office.

Nozick, R. 1974. *Anarchy, State, and Utopia.* New York: Basic Books.

Outka, G. 1975. "Social Justice and Equal Access to Health Care." *Perspectives in Biology and Medicine* 18: 185–203.

Rawls, J. 1971. *A Theory of Justice.* Cambridge: Harvard University Press.

Roemer, M. 1985. "I. S. Falk, the Committee on the Costs of Medical Care, and the Drive for National Health Insurance." *American Journal of Public Health* 75: 841–48.

Rosenblatt, R. 1989. "The Perinatal Paradox." *Health Affairs* 8 (September): 158–68.

Sager, M., D. Easterling, D. Kindig, and O. Anderson. 1989. "Changes in the Location of Death after Passage of Medicare's Prospective Payment System." *New England Journal of Medicine* 320: 433–39.

Singer, I., A. Meyerhoff, and S. Schiffman. 1985. *A Guide to Health Data Resources.* Millwood, VA: Project HOPE, Center for Health Affairs.

Stewart, A., S. Greenfield, R. Hays, K. Wells, W. Rogers, S. Berry, E. McGlynn, and J. Ware. 1989. "Functional Status and Well-being of Patients with Chronic Conditions: Results from the Medical Outcomes Study." *Journal of the American Medical Association* 262: 907–13.

Torrance, G. W. 1986. "Measurement of Health State Utilities for Economic Appraisal—A Review." *Journal of Health Economics* 5: 1–30.

Veatch, R. 1981. *A Theory of Medical Ethics.* New York: Basic Books.

Ware, J., and M. Synder. 1975. "Dimensions of Patient Attitudes Regarding Doctor and Medical Care Services." *Medical Care* 13: 669–82.

Wood, J., and C. Estes. 1990. "The Impact of DRGs on Community-based Service Providers: Implications for the Elderly." *American Journal of Public Health* 80: 840–43.

Equity of Access: Evidence
and an Application

This chapter summarizes the evidence on the extent to which the goal of equity of access to medical care has been achieved in the United States and reviews how universal health insurance might contribute to furthering this objective. Findings from health services research regarding the correlates and indicators of equity discussed in Chapter 6 are presented. The contributions of universal health insurance (UHI) and the criteria for evaluating UHI proposals in terms of the equity objective are introduced in this chapter, and Chapter 9 applies them to selected UHI alternatives.

Evidence Relating to Equity
of Access to Medical Care

The following discussion examines the findings from descriptive, analytic, and evaluative health services research on equity of access to medical care to address the major question posed in this chapter, how well has the U.S. medical care system achieved its goal to provide the freedom and equality of opportunity to obtain adequate and effective medical care? The answer, based on available evidence, is "not very well."

A plethora of social indicator–type measures have been utilized to document the performance of the U.S. medical care system with respect to equity. Illustrative examples and estimates of indicators of this objective, provided in Table 6.2, are detailed in Appendix 7.1. However, the presentation and discussion of findings focus principally on trends in potential access indicators and their relationship to predicting people's actual utilization and levels of satisfaction with medical care.

Characteristics of the delivery system

Availability

Potential access. The major policy concerns regarding the availability of medical care personnel and resources in an area have shifted over the past 30 years from the issue of *how many* providers there are to *where* the providers are located and *who* exactly is being served. The distribution of providers and, more important, the effect of service availability on whether or not care is sought, have been and continue to be a focus of health policy efforts regarding access.

Post–World War II policies to support the training of medical personnel and new hospital construction led to overall increases in the number of providers and facilities. These increases were mirrored in steady rises in the traditional provider- and facility-to-population ratios. The number of active physicians per 10,000 population, for example, increased around two-thirds, from 14.1 in 1950 to 22.3 in 1989 (NCHS 1992, 245). The number of hospital beds per 1,000 civilian population expanded by over a third, from 3.2 in 1940 to a high of 4.5 in 1980, though it has declined in recent years—to 3.8 in 1989 (NCHS 1992, 258–59).

Wide variability exists in the geographic distribution of providers. In 1989 the number of active nonfederal physicians per 10,000 civilian population ranged from 58.0 in Washington, D.C. to 14.2 in Alaska, and the South had the fewest nurses (562.2) and dentists (46.8) per 100,000 resident population of any region (NCHS 1990c; 1992, 243–44, 247).

A related issue of availability, however, is whether providers are willing to see patients who have public insurance or who are uninsured. The overall proportion of physicians refusing to see Medicaid clients declined from 22.7 percent in 1977–78 to 16.5 percent in 1984–85. A similar decline occurred for obstetrician-gynecologists: from 35.6 percent to 27.1 percent. Nonetheless, physician refusal to see Medicaid clients creates a significant barrier to care for low-income, pregnant women—particularly those residing in heavily minority inner-city areas (Mitchell 1991).

Actual access. Research during the 1970s and early 1980s suggested that provider-to-population ratios alone did not determine actual rates of use. Even in areas of ostensible shortage, residents with transportation and financial resources traveled out of the neighborhood or to adjoining towns for care (Chiu, Aday, and Andersen 1981; Kleinman and Wilson 1977).

There has, however, been heightened concern over the effect of a number of trends at the national and local level on the availability of providers, as well as the resultant utilization patterns of residents, in rural and inner-city communities. These include an increase in the rates of closure of rural hospitals and financially stressed urban hospitals serving poor, inner-city populations; primary care provider flight from or reluctance to locate in these same areas; and a large proportion of physicians in certain specialties (such as obstetrics-gynecology) who have closed their practices to medically indigent and Medicaid patients, due to the low rates of public third-party reimbursement and heightened fears of medical malpractice liability (Aiken and Mullinix 1987; Bureau of Health Professions 1990; Ermann 1990; Frenzen 1991; General Accounting Office 1990, 1991; *Health Services Research* 1989; Iglehart 1987; Institute of Medicine 1989a, 1989b; Kindig and Movassaghi 1989; Mullner et al. 1989; National Commission to Prevent Infant Mortality 1988; Office of Technology Assessment 1990; Schloss 1988; Schwartz, Sloan, and Mendelson 1988; United States Congress 1988).

The effect of these changes on actual patterns of service use depends to a large extent on whether alternative service delivery arrangements subsequently become available to the populations previously served by these providers (e.g., through reconfiguring a formerly inpatient-oriented rural hospital to a primary care or emergency care service provider). The lack of an adequate system of primary care in general, and maternity and prenatal care services in particular, for low-income, inner-city women and poor and ethnic minorities living in isolated rural counties or communities (such as along the Texas-Mexico border) has been found to contribute to their lower rates of use of preventive, as well as illness-related, care (Fossett et al. 1990; Institute of Medicine 1988; Warner 1991).

Organization

Potential access. The organization and financing of medical care in the United States increasingly reflect a multiple-tiered system of service provision for the privately insured middle and upper class, the elderly who have Medicare only, the Medicaid-eligible indigent or working-class poor population, and individuals and families with neither public nor private coverage. Such divisions have, in some sense, always been a fact of life in the U.S. medical care system. They emerge as a particular paradox now, however, because as the overall public and private commitment of expenditures for medical care continues to rise, so does the number of Americans who have no or inadequate protection against these burgeoning increases.

Relman (1980) has characterized the emerging U.S. "medical-industrial complex" as a large and growing network of private corporations engaged in the business of supplying medical care to patients for a profit, such as chain hospitals, emergicenters, walk-in clinics, dialysis centers, and home health care companies. The diverse and evolving forms of private medical practice are also increasingly linked to methods of paying for care. These include group practice–based health maintenance organizations, individual practice associations (IPAs), preferred provider organizations, and managed care organizations (MCOs), among others. The organizational distinctions between these different arrangements are becoming increasingly obscure. All of these alternatives have attempted to develop systems of cost-conscious medical practice and methods of reimbursement (Feldman, Kralewski, and Dowd 1989; Morrison and Luft 1990).

The number of health maintenance organizations (group and IPA models) increased from 174 in 1976 to a peak of 647 in 1987. Though the total enrollment in such plans has continued to grow, the number of plans has diminished since then (to 553 in 1991), primarily due to mergers and closures as a result of increased competition (NCHS 1992, 293).

The growing number of elderly (particularly the oldest old) and the impetus for shortened lengths of hospital stays resulting from DRGs have put increasing pressures on nursing homes. The number of nursing home beds per 1,000 resident population 85 years of age and over declined from 681.4 in 1976 to 582.2 in 1986 (NCHS 1992, 264–65).

The deinstitutionalization movement in mental health care led to the discharge of large numbers of the mentally ill into the community and a greatly diminished emphasis on long-term inpatient care. For example, the number of inpatient residential and treatment beds in mental health organizations per 100,000 civilian population dropped from 263.6 in 1970 to 111.5 in 1988 (NCHS 1992, 257).

Actual access. The major concerns underlying the actual access impact of this increasing corporatization of medical practice relate to the fact that private and for-profit institutions are less likely to serve the poor and medically indigent, and that large-scale bureaucratic, publicly supported providers are less likely to be convenient and satisfactory to consumers (Aday 1987).

The poor and elderly have, for example, generally been underrepresented in HMO and private insurance plans, principally because such plans have tended to enroll the employed and their dependents, the vast majority of whom are under 65 and not poor. Demonstration projects and programs, supported by the Health Care Financing Administration, to enroll the poor and elderly in such arrangements have met with mixed success in terms of access, cost, and quality objectives.

In general, enrollees expressed less satisfaction with providers than patients at comparison sites (Freund et al. 1989; Langwell and Hadley 1989). The RAND Health Insurance Experiment documented lower client satisfaction among HMO enrollees compared to fee-for-service clients (Wagner and Bledsoe 1990; Ware et al. 1986), and a more recent RAND evaluation of PPOs demonstrated that PPO enrollees were also generally more satisfied than those in HMOs (Hosek et al. 1990).

There is evidence that both nonprofit and for-profit, *private* institutions are less willing to serve patients without insurance, and have much lower rates of uncompensated and undercompensated care, than do publicly supported, teaching hospitals in particular (Gray 1986; Sloan, Blumstein, and Perrin 1986). Users of publicly supported facilities (such as public health clinics and hospital outpatient departments or emergency rooms) may often have to wait hours to be seen when they or ill or injured or may be told it will be weeks or even months before they can get an appointment for a routine or prevention-related visit (for prenatal care, for example) (Freeman et al. 1987; Institute of Medicine 1988; Robert Wood Johnson Foundation 1987; Tavani 1991).

Financing

Potential access. The advent of Medicaid and Medicare in the mid-1960s led to a significant increase in the percentage of health services and supplies (HSS) (that is, the cost of health care excluding research and construction) paid for by the federal government, from 9 percent in 1965 to 18 percent in 1980. Private businesses also assumed a larger role in financing health care through employer-based coverage. The percentage of HSS expenditures by private businesses increased from 17 percent in 1965 to 27 percent in 1980, while the proportion of expenditures borne by households or individuals declined from 61 percent to 38 percent over this same period (Levit and Cowan 1991). In 1990, each of the major components paid for approximately one-third of the nation's health care costs: 33 percent of the expenditures were from public sources (including 18 percent from the federal government and 15 percent from state and local governments); 29 percent from private businesses; 35 percent from individuals; and 3 percent from nonpatient revenues (philanthropic funds, providers' interest income, and so on).

During the past decade, as the costs of care continued to rise, there was an increasing interest on the part of public and private third-party payers in reducing the amounts they had to pay for medical care. They have, therefore, imposed stricter eligibility criteria; cutbacks in covered services; fixed, predetermined (prospective) rates of reimbursement by service or diagnosis (such as DRGs); and greater consumer cost sharing. Expenditures for health services and supplies as a percentage of household (or individual income), which remained relatively stable from 1965 to 1980 (around 4.2 percent), rose steadily to 5.0 percent in 1990 (Levit and Cowan 1991).

Actual access. Empirical findings related to the major prospective pricing initiative in recent years (reimbursement for hospital services under Medicare on the basis of DRGs) on hospital utilization and expenditures show that admission rates, total days of care, and average length of stay have declined since its introduction. These trends are, however, confounded with trends that were already underway in the organization and delivery of medical care prior to the introduction of DRGs (such as an increased emphasis on ambulatory care) (Edwards and Gibson 1990; *Health Care Financing Review* 1989; Russell and Manning 1989; Sloan, Morrisey, and Valvona 1988).

Nonetheless, there is evidence in many communities that the elderly were being discharged after shorter stays and in poorer health, largely as a result of providers' responses to the DRG pricing policy. The post-discharge death rates for those in unstable condition were higher after the introduction of DRGs—particularly among those discharged home rather than to a nursing home or other institutional care setting (Kosecoff et al. 1990). The tendency to discharge such patients when they reach the limit of reimbursable days has also exposed deficiencies in the posthospitalization system of care for the chronically ill and elderly in many communities, such as inadequate discharge planning, an insufficient number of nursing home beds, lack of community support services, and corollary stresses on the patient's family and other caregivers (Gornick and Hall 1988; Kenney and Holahan 1991).

Medicaid, which was set up initially to provide coverage for the medically indigent, is now the principal payer of long-term care (particularly nursing home services) for the elderly (Oberg and Polich 1988). Major cutbacks in the Medicaid program during the early 1980s resulted in dramatic reductions in the number of individuals and scope of services covered in many states, which federally mandated expansions of coverage to categories of the poor during the middle to late 1980s attempted to redress (Holahan and Zedlewski 1991; Johns and Adler 1989).

The RAND Health Insurance Experiment (HIE) documented an inverse relationship between the amount of physician and hospital services consumed and the amount of consumer copayment—the more consumers had to pay, the less medical care they consumed. The office-based medical use rates for children were particularly likely to be lower for those in cost-sharing compared to free care plans (Anderson, Brook, and

Williams 1991). Though the HIE documented minimal negative health consequences overall as a result of plan cost-sharing provisions, the effects that were found were primarily among low-income, chronically ill individuals (Lohr et al. 1986). Medical care expenses tend to represent a much higher proportion of the total income of low-income families than is the case for higher-income families. Policies that encourage greater cost sharing by consumers will undoubtedly lower the overall use of services. The resultant economic and health effects are, however, most likely to fall on the poorest and sickest.

Characteristics of the population

The focus in reviewing evidence with respect to equity in terms of the characteristics of the population is the effect of an array of predisposing, enabling, and need factors on the population's use of and satisfaction with medical care.

Predisposing

Age is significantly associated with all different types of medical care service use, primarily because it is an important indicator of age-associated morbidity. Women use more health services than do men in general, which is to a varying extent a function of their obstetrics-related care needs, greater longevity, and the fact that it is perceived more socially acceptable for women to engage in help-seeking behaviors (Aday 1992). As noted earlier, however, substantial availability, organizational, and financial barriers exist for categories of women (especially low-income, uninsured, or Medicaid-eligible women) seeking prenatal and maternity care services.

Education is an important predictor of the use of preventive services. Better-educated people are, for example, more likely to have had a general physical, immunizations, tests, and procedures for preventive purposes and better-educated women are more likely to have sought care early in their pregnancy (Aday and Eichhorn 1972; Maurana, Eichhorn, and Lonnquist 1981; NCHS 1988, 1990a, 1991a, 1991b).

The influence of these predisposing factors on utilization has remained relatively stable over time.

Enabling

According to the 1987 National Medical Expenditure Survey (NMES), 18.8 percent of the population did not have a usual source of care. Among those who did, a physician's office was used most frequently (85.7 percent), followed by health centers and sites such as company or school clinics (8.0 percent), and hospital outpatient departments or emergency rooms (6.3 percent). Blacks, Hispanics, the poor, males, adults aged 19 to 24, residents of large metropolitan statistical areas, and the uninsured were least likely to have a regular source of care and, among those who did, to use a hospital outpatient department or emergency room (Cornelius, Beauregard, and Cohen 1991).

The number of Americans lacking either public or private insurance on any given day has been estimated to range from 31 to 37 million. The number uninsured at some time (all or part) of the year is estimated to be even higher (around 48 million) (Friedman 1991). The 1987 NMES found that those most likely to be uninsured at some point during the year were young adults and children under 18; Hispanics and blacks; and the poor (Short 1990). The percentage under 65 who were uninsured at the time of the 1989 National Center for Health Statistics Health Interview Survey was much higher for blacks (20.2 percent) and other nonwhite individuals (19.7 percent) than for whites (12.8 percent); for the poor (32.5 percent) than for those who were not poor (10.3 percent); and for the unemployed (38.3 percent) than for those who were working (13.9 percent) (Ries 1991).

According to the 1987 NMES, the vast majority of uninsured (77 percent) were in families with a working adult. The employed uninsured were more likely to work part-time (24 percent) or be self-employed (23 percent); to work in construction (30 percent) or service industries (31 percent); not to be in a union (16 percent); to work in small firms with less than ten workers (26 percent); and to be earning less than $5.00 an hour (30 percent) (Short, Monheit, and Beauregard 1989).

Further, around one in four (26 percent) of the nonelderly insured have been estimated to be underinsured or "inadequately protected against the possibility of large medical bills" (Farley 1985).

The proportion of the poor and near-poor covered by Medicaid reached a peak of 64 percent in the mid-1970s and subsequently declined to around 40 percent in the mid- to late 1980s. Recent Medicaid expansions have attempted to reverse this trend, particularly for low-income women, infants and children (Friedman 1991).

Need

Assessments of need may be based on patients' self-perceptions of their health, as well as on medical professionals' clinical diagnoses and evaluations. Providers' and patients' evaluations of needs may not always agree. Nonetheless, need, however measured, is consistently borne out to be an important predictor of the use of services—particularly the volume of services consumed. (See the discussion of use relative to need that follows.) Need is, for example, generally the most important predictor of the number of physician visits for those with at least one visit, and of the number of days of care, once a patient is admitted to the hospital. For more preventive-oriented or discretionary services, such as dental care, need has been and continues to be less important than other (particularly enabling) factors (such as income or insurance coverage) (Aday, Andersen, and Fleming 1980; Andersen et al. 1987).

Utilization

Race, income, having a regular source of care, and insurance coverage are important policy-relevant predictors of the utilization of medical care services.

Despite improvements in the levels of access to medical care among Hispanics, blacks, and other minorities, they are still less likely to use certain types of services than are whites. Mexican-Americans in particular are less apt to have seen a physician or dentist or to have been hospitalized than are whites, blacks, or other categories of Hispanics. Hispanic and Native American women are less likely to have sought caring during the first trimester or, in some cases, at all during their pregnancy. The lack of insurance coverage appears to be a particularly important contributor to Hispanics' lower use of medical and dental services (Andersen, Giachello, and Aday 1986; Ginzberg 1991; NCHS 1984; 1992; Trevino et al. 1991).

The proportion of women seeking care in the first trimester of their pregnancy, preschool children who are immunized, or adults or children who have been to a dentist is much lower among African-Americans than among whites. The incidence of congenital syphilis and late-stage cancer, which could have been prevented through early intervention, is also higher among African-Americans (Manton, Patrick, and Johnson 1987; NCHS 1990b, 1992).

In the past, people with higher incomes used more medical care services than those with lower incomes. With the enactment of Medicare and Medicaid, the rates of utilization increased greatly among the poor. Nonetheless, income-related use differentials remain. The rates of use of physician and hospital services in general relative to need are lower for the poor—particularly the poor or working poor who have no insurance.

In 1990, the percentage seeing a doctor in the year was lower for people from families with incomes less than $14,000 (77.3 percent), than for those with family incomes of $50,000 or more (81.7 percent). People with lower incomes were nonetheless in much poorer health than people with higher incomes, based on subjective perceptions of health, reported days of limited activity due to illness, and limitations in major activity due to the presence of a chronic condition. Since the introduction of Medicaid and Medicare, the rates of hospital discharges, days of care, and length of stay, and the mean number of visits to a physician, once seen, have tended to be higher for those with lower, compared to those with higher, incomes—reflecting perhaps their greater need, as well as their greater tendency to delay seeking care, until the health problem has worsened (NCHS 1992, 200, 202, 219, 220).

Having a regular source of medical care is a strong and consistent predictor of medical care utilization, particularly for whether care is sought initially. Once entry is gained, having an established provider is less significant in predicting the subsequent number of visits to a physician or the length of time in the hospital (Andersen et al. 1987). Questions have been raised about the accuracy of self-reports of usual source of care, as well as whether having a regular source of care is a determinant or a result of using services (Perloff and Morris 1989). Causal models testing the direction of this relationship have confirmed that having an identifiable medical provider does directly influence the decision of whether or not to seek care (Kuder and Levitz 1985).

The presence and extent of insurance coverage have been demonstrated to be important predictors of the utilization of medical care services in numerous national and local studies of access (Andersen et al. 1987; Davis and Rowland 1983; Freeman et al. 1990; Kasper 1986; Rosenbach 1989; Wilensky and Berk 1982). There is, in addition, growing evidence that patients with private third-party coverage are more likely to receive more intensive and technology-oriented care than those with public coverage or no insurance (Hadley, Steinberg, and Feder 1991; Wenneker, Weissman, and Epstein 1990). Studies in states that have dropped large numbers of the poor from the Medicaid program have shown corollary increases in adverse health outcomes, such as higher infant mortality rates (Braveman et al. 1989).

Satisfaction

Surveys of public and patient opinion regarding the performance of the medical care system in different countries confirm that U.S. residents are much more critical of the system as a whole and much less satisfied with their own particular experiences in getting care than are people in other countries, such as Canada and the United Kingdom. Only 10 percent of U.S residents thought that the health care system worked pretty well and that only minor changes were needed, in contrast to 56 percent of Canadians and 27 percent of United Kingdom residents.

Similarly, 57 percent of U.S. residents who had been hospitalized were very satisfied with their stay, compared to 71 percent in Canada and 67 percent in the United Kingdom. The percentages of patients who were very satisfied with visits to their physician were 54 percent in the United States, 73 percent in Canada, and 63 percent in the United Kingdom (Blendon and Taylor 1989).

Summary

An array of indicators of the performance of the U.S. medical care system in terms of equity suggest that it falls short of achieving this goal. A particular challenge to descriptive health services research in developing indicators of the adequacy of access to medical care is to identify the domains of need (including risks or conditions) for which medical care could make a difference. In addition, analytic and evaluative health services research is needed to assess the probable or actual effect of different ways of financing (such as alternative physician and hospital payment systems) and delivering care (health maintenance organizations, preferred providers, or other managed care options) on access to care.

An Application: Universal Health Insurance Proposals

The access problem

As indicated in the previous discussion, people with insurance generally have better access to care than those who do not. Holes that have appeared in the safety net of public and private coverage during the past decade have led to the access problem being principally defined as an issue of the number of uninsured and underinsured Americans. This definition of the access problem has given rise to an energetic debate at the national level regarding alternative means to address the "insurance problem."

The increasing number of uninsured and underinsured Americans is due to the erosion of coverage under both public and private insurance programs. Medicare beneficiaries' out-of-pocket costs of care have continued to increase, and coverage for long-term care under this program remains inadequate.

The withdrawal of federal support has been greatest for the Medicaid program. Due to the cutbacks enacted in the Medicaid program in the 1980s, the number of beneficiaries remained stable during a period in which the number of poor continued to grow. Because of the categoric eligibility requirements for Medicaid (through Aid to Families with Dependent Children (AFDC) or Supplementary Security Income, for example), certain groups of the poor, such as nondisabled men and childless couples, do not qualify, regardless of income. In the late 1980s, Congress mandated Medicaid coverage for low-income pregnant women and young children—a move that many states resisted because of the substantial increase in funding required. Though AFDC families make up 70 percent to 75 percent of the Medicaid population, a similar percentage of Medicaid expenditures goes to paying for the care of a *different* group of eligibles—the aged, blind, and disabled in nursing homes. The net effect of these paradoxes in the Medicaid program for the poor is that it leaves out more poor Americans (60 percent) than it covers (40 percent).

Comparable erosions have occurred in the coverage available to employed people and their dependents through the workplace. A major element in the crisis of the uninsured is the increasing cost of medical care, which many businesses, particularly small employers, are not able to afford. The adaptations that employers have made in response—limiting coverage of dependents, using experience rating, refusing to cover those deemed "uninsurable," canceling policies on short notice, and raising premiums—have also served to reduce the availability of coverage to employed persons and their dependents (Friedman 1991).

Alternative solutions

The policy debate regarding "access" has correspondingly focused on developing alternatives for more universal methods of coverage. Two assumptions underlying this perspective are that getting medical care helps to improve one's health, and that no one, because of inability to pay the doctor or hospital, should be denied care.

These assumptions, however, sidestep questions of whether values or objectives other than equity (however defined), are at the heart of the "access" problem. Is the intent of expanded coverage to assure patients better access to needed services or to assure that someone pays the bills for the expensive and, in some instances, marginally effective, high-technology, intensive, clinically oriented care? Whose interests are served by this coverage—providers' or patients'? Does access to medical care necessarily mean access to better health, or is it really fairer to spend societal resources in other ways to ensure *that* outcome?

A variety of factors have contributed to the accelerated levels of spending for medical care. These include, among others, that one of the extremely costly compromises struck with the organized medical com-munity to assure the passage of Medicare and Medicaid in the mid-1960s was *not* to interfere with the fee-for-service method of reimbursing physicians. The resultant policy of paying physicians their "usual and customary" fee opened a spigot of expenditures for high-technology, in-tensive, expensive, acute-oriented medical care that federal policy efforts have only recently begun to try to staunch. Designing new mechanisms for paying for basically the same, high-priced style of U.S. medical care practice may not be either the most effective, the most efficient, or the most equitable use of finite societal resources. The physician payment and outcomes management proposals discussed in previous chapters represent attempts to address this important and corollary dimension of the access problem, implicit in proposals to reform the system of paying for medical care.

The evidence presented earlier regarding access also suggests that reducing or eliminating the financial barriers will not necessarily *solve* the access problem. The system of services for poor, minority, inner-city, and rural populations, as well as a variety of other categories of vulnerable populations (high-risk mothers and infants, persons with AIDS, drug users, and victims of family abuse, among others), remains fragmented, inconvenient, and inadequate. For these groups, at least, the goal of achieving financial access still poses the question, to what will they *have* access?

Development of universal health insurance proposals

A plethora of proposals for more-universal methods of financing medical care have emerged in recent years, sponsored by a variety of constituen-cies (physician associations, employer coalitions, and organized labor, among others). They all attempt to enhance near-universal coverage for services, but differ primarily in the means for doing so (Blendon and Edwards 1991).

The proposals may be grouped into three major types: (1) reform-oriented, *private market–based* proposals to create a more cost-efficient array of alternatives for people to purchase coverage; (2) *employer-based* ("play or pay") proposals that build on the present system, whereby employers either provide insurance to employees or pay taxes to fi-nance an alternative public system; and (3) reform-oriented, *government-sponsored, single-payer* plans modeled primarily on the Canadian system. Individual states are also experimenting with options for extending more universal coverage (General Accounting Office 1992). The Clinton admin-istration has expressed an interest in models of managed competition with expenditure limits, which would combine elements of each of these proposals.

The final question addressed in this chapter is, will universal health insurance assist in achieving the goal of providing the freedom and equality of opportunity to obtain adequate and effective medical care? The answer offered here is that whether or not universal health insurance promotes that goal depends on the plan.

Criteria of equity for evaluating universal health insurance proposals

Three plans that illustrate the three primary models for reform will be reviewed here and in Chapter 9. These include the Consumer Choice Health Plan (CCHP), the National Health Program (NHP) proposed by Physicians for a National Health Program, and the Pepper Commission proposal (PCP). Enthoven and Kronick's managed competition proposal, the CCHP, has elements of a play-or-pay strategy. However, its primary focus is the development of procompetitive medical care markets within states (Enthoven and Kronick 1989a, 1989b, 1991). The National Health Program is a market-minimized alternative, modeled to a considerable extent after the Canadian system (Grumbach et al. 1991; Himmelstein et al. 1989). The Pepper Commission proposal is a mixed plan that builds most directly on the features of the current system of employer-based private coverage, but also suggests changes to address a number of existing sources of inequity (Pepper Commission 1990; Rockefeller 1991). None of these proposals is likely to be adopted in its entirety. These alternatives do, however, provide an opportunity to analyze the components of competing models, and their probable contribution to the equity objective.

Appendix 7.2 summarizes the criteria that will serve as the basis for evaluating the extent to which the features of selected plans are likely to enhance equity of access to medical care. Chapter 9 reviews and critiques examples of each of the three major types of plans with respect to their probable contribution to the equity, as well as effectiveness and efficiency, objectives.

The major question with which this chapter began was, how well has the U.S. medical care system achieved its goal of equity of access to medical care? The answer offered here is, "not very well." The success of health services researchers concerned with understanding whether universal health insurance will assist in enhancing equity of access to medical care requires the full partnership of researchers committed to clarifying and evaluating the effectiveness and efficiency objectives as well.

References

Aday, L. 1987. "The Ethical Implications of Prospective Payment and Corporate Medical Practice: A Research Agenda." *Social Justice Research* 1: 275–96.

———. 1992. "Indicators and Predictors of Health Services Utilization." In *Introduction to Health Services*, edited by Stephen J. Williams and Paul R. Torrens. New York: John Wiley & Sons.

Aday, L., R. Andersen, and G. Fleming. 1980. *Health Care in the U.S.: Equitable for Whom?* Beverly Hills: Sage Publications.

Aday, L., and R. Eichhorn. 1972. *The Utilization of Health Services: Indices and Correlates—A Research Bibliography.* DHEW Pub. No. (HSM) 73-3003. Washington, DC: U.S. Government Printing Office.

Aiken, L., and C. Mullinix. 1987. "Special Report: The Nurse Shortage—Myth or Reality? *New England Journal of Medicine* 317: 641–46.

Andersen, R., L. Aday, C. Lyttle, L. Cornelius, and M. Chen. 1987. *Ambulatory Care and Insurance Coverage in an Era of Constraint.* Chicago: Pluribus Press, Inc.

Andersen, R., A. Giachello, and L. Aday. 1986. "Access of Hispanics to Health Care and Cuts in Services: A State of the Art Overview." *Public Health Reports* 101: 238–52.

Anderson, G., R. Brook, and A. Williams. 1991. "A Comparison of Cost-Sharing versus Free Care in Children: Effects on the Demand for Office-based Medical Care." *Medical Care* 29: 890–98.

Blendon, R., and J. Edwards. 1991. "Caring for the Uninsured: Choices for Reform." *Journal of the American Medical Association* 265: 2563–65.

Blendon, R., and H. Taylor. 1989. "Views on Health Care: Public Opinion in Three Nations." *Health Affairs* 8 (March): 149–57.

Braveman, P., G. Oliva, M. Miller, R. Reiter, and S. Egerter. 1989. "Adverse Outcomes and Lack of Health Insurance among Newborns in an Eight-County Area of California, 1982 to 1986." *New England Journal of Medicine* 321: 508–13.

Bureau of Health Professions. 1990. *Seventh Report to the Congress on the Status of Health Personnel in the United States.* Rockville, MD: Health Resources and Services Administration.

Chiu, G., L. Aday, and R. Andersen. 1981. "An Examination of the Association of 'Shortage' and 'Medical Access' Indicators." *Health Policy Quarterly* 1: 142–58.

Cornelius, L., K. Beauregard, and J. Cohen. 1991. *Usual Sources of Medical Care and Their Characteristics.* AHCPR Pub. No. 91-0042, National Medical Expenditure Survey Research Findings 11. Rockville, MD: Agency for Health Care Policy and Research.

Davis, K., and D. Rowland. 1983. "Uninsured and Underserved: Inequities in Health Care in the United States." *Milbank Memorial Fund Quarterly/Health and Society* 61: 149–76.

Edwards, W., and D. Gibson. 1990. "Geographic Variations in Medicare Utilization of Short-Stay Hospital Services, 1981–88." *Health Care Financing Review* 11 (March): 107–11.

Enthoven, A., and R. Kronick. 1989a. "A Consumer-Choice Health Plan for the 1990s: Universal Health Insurance in a System Designed to Promote Quality and Economy." *New England Journal of Medicine* 320: 29–37.

———. 1989b. "A Consumer-Choice Health Plan for the 1990s: Universal Health Insurance in a System Designed to Promote Quality and Economy." *New England Journal of Medicine* 320: 94–101.

———. 1991. "Universal Health Insurance through Incentives Reform." *Journal of the American Medical Association* 265: 2532–36.

Ermann, D. 1990. "Rural Health Care: The Future of the Hospital." *Medical Care Review* 47: 33–73.

Farley, P. 1985. "Who Are the Underinsured?" *Milbank Memorial Fund Quarterly/Health and Society* 63: 476–503.

Feldman, R., J. Kralewski, and B. Dowd. 1989. "Health Maintenance Organizations: The Beginning or the End?" *Health Services Research* 24: 191–211.

Fossett, J., J. Perloff, J. Peterson, and P. Kletke. 1990. "Medicaid in the Inner City: The Case of Maternity Care in Chicago." *Milbank Quarterly* 68: 111–41.

Freeman, H., L. Aiken, R. Blendon, and C. Corey. 1990. "Uninsured Working-Age Adults: Characteristics and Consequences." *Health Services Research* 24: 811–23.

Freeman, H., R. Blendon, L. Aiken, S. Sudman, C. Mullinix, and C. Corey. 1987. "Americans Report on Their Access to Health Care." *Health Affairs* 6 (March): 6–18.

Frenzen, P. 1991. "The Increasing Supply of Physicians in U.S. Urban and Rural Areas, 1975 to 1988." *American Journal of Public Health* 81: 1141–47.

Freund, D., L. Rossiter, P. Fox, J. Meyer, R. Hurley, T. Carey, and J. Paul. 1989. "Evaluation of the Medicaid Competition Demonstrations." *Health Care Financing Review* 11 (December): 81–97.

Friedman, E. 1991. "The Uninsured: From Dilemma to Crisis." *Journal of the American Medical Association* 265: 2491–95.

General Accounting Office. 1990. *National Health Services Corps Program Unable to Meet Need for Physicians in Underserved Areas.* GAO/HRD-90-128. Washington, DC: U.S. General Accounting Office.

———. 1991. *Rural Hospitals: Federal Efforts Should Target Areas Where Closures Would Threaten Access to Care.* GAO/HRD-91-41. Washington, DC: U.S. General Accounting Office.

———. 1992. *Access to Health Care: States Respond to Growing Crisis.* GAO/HRD-92-70. Washington, DC: U.S. General Accounting Office.

Ginzberg, E. 1991. "Access to Health Care for Hispanics." *Journal of the American Medical Association* 265: 238–41.

Gornick, M., and M. Hall. 1988. "Trends in Medicare Use of Post-hospital Care." *Health Care Financing Review, Annual Supplement:* 27–38.

Gray, B. H. 1986. *For-Profit Enterprise in Health Care.* Washington, DC: National Academy Press.

Grumbach, K., T. Bodenheimer, D. Himmelstein, and S. Woolhandler. 1991. "Liberal Benefits, Conservative Spending: The Physicians for a National Health Program Proposal." *Journal of the American Medical Association* 265: 2549–54.

Hadley, J., E. Steinberg, and J. Feder. 1991. "Comparison of Uninsured and Privately Insured Hospital Patients." *Journal of the American Medical Association* 265: 374–79.

Health Care Financing Review. 1989. "The Impact of the Medicare Hospital Prospective Payment System: 1986 Annual Report." *Health Care Financing Review* 10 (March): 160–61.

Health Services Research. 1989. "Special Issue: A Rural Health Services Research Agenda." *Health Services Research* 23: 725–1083.

Himmelstein, D., S. Woolhandler, and the Writing Committee of the Working Group on Program Design. 1989. "A National Health Program for the United States: A Physicians' Proposal." *New England Journal of Medicine* 320: 102–8.

Holahan, J., and S. Zedlewski. 1991. "Expanding Medicaid to Cover Uninsured Americans." *Health Affairs* 10 (March): 45–61.

Hosek, S., M. S. Marquis, K. Wells, D. Garnick, and H. Luft. 1990. *The Study of Preferred Provider Organizations: Executive Summary.* R-3798-HHS/NIMH. Santa Monica, CA: RAND Corporation.

Iglehart, J. 1987. "Health Policy Report: Problems Facing the Nursing Profession." *New England Journal of Medicine* 317: 646–51.

Institute of Medicine. 1988. *Prenatal Care: Reaching Mothers, Reaching Infants.* Washington, DC: National Academy Press.

———. 1989a. *Medical Professional Liability and the Delivery of Obstetrical Care, Volume I.* Washington, DC: National Academy Press.

———. 1989b. *Medical Professional Liability and the Delivery of Obstetrical Care, Volume II.* Washington, DC: National Academy Press.

Johns, L., and G. Adler. 1989. "Evaluation of Recent Changes in Medicaid." *Health Affairs* 8 (March): 171–81.

Kasper, J. 1986. "Health Status and Utilization: Differences by Medicaid Coverage and Income." *Health Care Financing Review* 7 (June): 1–17.

Kenney, G., and J. Holahan. 1991. "Nursing Home Transfers and Mean Length of Stay in the Prospective Payment Era." *Medical Care* 29: 589–609.

Kindig, D., and H. Movassaghi. 1989. "The Adequacy of Physician Supply in Small Rural Counties." *Health Affairs* 8 (June): 63–76.

Kleinman, J., and R. Wilson. 1977. "Are the Medically Underserved Areas Medically Underserved?" *Health Services Research* 12: 147–62.

Kosecoff, J., K. Kahn, W. Rogers, E. Reinisch, M. Sherwood, L. Rubenstein, D. Draper, C. Roth, C. Chew, and R. Brook. 1990. "Prospective Payment System and Impairment at Discharge: The 'Quicker and Sicker' Story Revisited." *Journal of the American Medical Association* 264: 1980–83.

Kuder, J., and G. Levitz. 1985. "Visits to the Physician: An Evaluation of the Usual Source Effect." *Health Services Research* 20: 579–96.

Langwell, K., and J. Hadley. 1989. "Evaluation of the Medicare Competition Demonstrations." *Health Care Financing Review* 11 (December): 65–80.

Levit, K. R., and C. A. Cowan. 1991. "Business, Households, and Governments: Health Care Costs, 1990." *Health Care Financing Review* 13 (December): 83–93.

Lohr, K., R. Brook, C. Kamberg, G. Goldberg, A. Leibowitz, J. Kessey, D. Reboussin, and J. Newhouse. 1986. "Use of Medical Care in the RAND Health

Insurance Experiment: Diagnosis and Service-Specific Analyses in a Randomized Controlled Trial." *Medical Care* 24 (supp.): S1–87.

Manton, K., C. Patrick, and K. Johnson. 1987. "Health Differentials between Blacks and Whites: Recent Trends in Mortality and Morbidity." *Milbank Quarterly* 65 (supp. 1): 129–99.

Maurana, C., R. Eichhorn, and L. Lonnquist. 1981. *The Use of Health Services: Indices and Correlates—A Research Bibliography*. Rockville, MD: National Center for Health Services Research.

Mitchell, J. 1991. "Physician Participation in Medicaid Revisited." *Medical Care* 29: 645–53.

Morrison, E., and H. Luft. 1990. "Health Maintenance Organization Environments in the 1980s and Beyond." *Health Care Financing Review* 12 (September): 81–90.

Mullner, R., R. Rydman, D. Whiteis, and R. Rich. 1989. "Rural Community Hospitals and Factors Correlated with Their Risk of Closing." *Public Health Reports* 104: 315–25.

National Center for Health Statistics. 1984. *Health Indicators for Hispanic, Black, and White Americans*. DHHS Pub. No. PHS 84-1576. Washington, DC: U.S. Government Printing Office.

———. 1988. *Health Promotion and Disease Prevention, United States, 1985*. DHHS Pub. No. PHS 88-1591. Washington, DC: U.S. Government Printing Office.

———. 1990a. *Health, United States, 1989*. DHHS Pub. No. PHS 90-1232. Washington, DC: U.S. Government Printing Office.

———. 1990b. *Health of Black and White Americans, 1985–87*. DHHS Pub. No. PHS 90-1599. Washington, DC: U.S. Government Printing Office.

———. 1990c. *Breast Cancer Risk Factors and Screening: United States, 1987*. DHHS Pub. No. PHS 90-1500. Washington, DC: U.S. Government Printing Office.

———. 1991a. *Educational Differences in Health Status and Health Care*. DHHS Pub. No. PHS 91-1507. Washington, DC: U.S. Government Printing Office.

———. 1991b. *Health, United States, 1990*. DHHS Pub. No. PHS 91-1232. Washington, DC: U.S. Government Printing Office.

———. 1992. *Health, United States, 1991*. DHHS Pub. No. PHS 92-1232. Washington, DC: U.S. Government Printing Office.

National Commission to Prevent Infant Mortality. 1988. *Malpractice and Liability: An Obstetrical Crisis*. Washington, DC: National Commission to Prevent Infant Mortality.

Oberg, C., and C. Polich. 1988. "Medicaid: Entering the Third Decade." *Health Affairs* 7 (September): 83–96.

Office of Technology Assessment. 1990. *Health Care in Rural America*. OTA-H-435. Washington, DC: U.S. Government Printing Office.

Pepper Commission: U.S. Bipartisan Commission on Comprehensive Health Care. 1990. *A Call for Action: Final Report*. Washington, DC: U.S. Government Printing Office.

Perloff, J., and N. Morris. 1989. "Validating Reporting of Usual Sources of Health Care." In *Health Survey Research Methods*, edited by Floyd J. Fowler, Jr. DHHS

Publication No. PHS 89-3447. Washington, DC: U.S. Government Printing Office.

Relman, A. 1980. "The New Medical-Industrial Complex." *New England Journal of Medicine* 303: 963–70.

Ries, P. 1991. *Characteristics of Persons with and without Health Care Coverage: United States, 1989.* DHHS Pub. No. PHS 91-1250. Hyattsville, MD: National Center for Health Statistics.

Robert Wood Johnson Foundation. 1987. *Access to Health Care in the United States: Results of a 1986 Survey.* Special Report Number Two. Princeton, NJ: The Robert Wood Johnson Foundation.

Rockefeller, J. 1991. "A Call for Action: The Pepper Commissions's Blueprint for Health Care Reform." *Journal of the American Medical Association* 265: 2507–10.

Rosenbach, M. 1989. "The Impact of Medicaid on Physician Use by Low-income Children." *American Journal of Public Health* 79: 1220–26.

Russell, L., and C. Manning. 1989. "The Effect of Prospective Payment on Medicare Expenditures." *New England Journal of Medicine* 320: 439–44.

Schloss, E. 1988. "Sounding Board: Beyond GMENAC—Another Physician Shortage from 2010 to 2030?" *New England Journal of Medicine* 318: 920–22.

Schwartz, W., F. Sloan, and D. Mendelson. 1988. "Why There Will Be Little or No Physician Surplus between Now and the Year 2000." *New England Journal of Medicine* 318: 892–97.

Short, P. 1990. *Estimates of the Uninsured Population, Calendar Year 1987.* DHHS Publication No. PHS 90-3469. Rockville, MD: Agency for Health Care Policy and Research.

Short, P., A. Monheit, and K. Beauregard. 1989. *A Profile of Uninsured Americans.* DHHS Publication No. PHS 89-3443. Rockville, MD: National Center for Health Services Research and Health Care Technology Assessment.

Sloan, F., J. Blumstein, and J. Perrin. 1986. *Uncompensated Hospital Care: Rights and Responsibilities.* Baltimore: Johns Hopkins University Press.

Sloan, F., M. Morrisey, and J. Valvona. 1988. Effects of the Medicare Prospective Payment System on Hospital Cost Containment: An Early Appraisal." *Milbank Quarterly* 66: 191–220.

Tavani, C. 1991. "Report on a Seminar on Financing and Service Delivery: Issues in Caring for the Medically Underserved." *Public Health Reports* 106: 19–26.

Trevino, F., M. E. Moyer, R. B. Valdez, and C. Stroup-Benham. 1991. "Health Insurance Coverage and Utilization of Health Services by Mexican Americans, Mainland Puerto Ricans, and Cuban Americans." *Journal of the American Medical Association* 265: 233–37.

United States Congress, Senate Special Committee on Aging. 1988. *The Rural Health Care Challenge.* Serial No. 100-N. Washington, DC: U.S. Government Printing Office.

Wagner, E., and T. Bledsoe. 1990. "The RAND Health Insurance Experiment and HMOs." *Medical Care* 28: 191–200.

Ware, J., R. Brook, W. Rogers, E. Keeler, A. Ross-Davies, C. Sherbourne, G. Goldberg, P. Camp, and J. Newhouse. 1986. "Comparison of Health Outcomes at a Health Maintenance Organization with Those of Fee-for-Service Care." *Lancet* 1: 1017–22.

Warner, D. 1991. "Health Issues at the U.S.-Mexican Border." *Journal of the American Medical Association* 265: 242–47.

Wenneker, M., J. Weissman, and A. Epstein. 1990. "The Association of Payer with Utilization of Cardiac Procedures in Massachusetts." *Journal of the American Medical Association* 264: 1255–60.

Wilensky, G., and M. Berk. 1982. "Health Care, the Poor, and the Role of Medicaid." *Health Affairs* 1 (September): 93–100.

Appendix 7.1   Highlights of Selected Indicators of Equity of Access to Medical Care

Potential Access

Characteristics of the Delivery System

Availability: Distribution of providers (Mitchell 1991; NCHS 1990c, 1992)

Active nonfederal physicians per 10,000 civilian population (1989):
U.S. = 21.9; DC = 58.0; Texas = 17.8; Alaska = 14.2.

Registered nurses per 100,000 resident population (1989):
U.S. = 671.0; Northeast = 843.7; Midwest = 729.5; South = 562.2; West = 613.8.

Dentists per 100,000 resident population (1987):
U.S. = 57.8; Northeast = 69.3; Midwest = 60.7; South = 46.8; West = 61.0.

Percentage of physicians refusing to see Medicaid patients:	*1977–78*	*1984–85*
— Total physicians	22.7%	16.5%
— Obstetrician-gynecologists	35.6	27.1

Organization: Types of facilities (NCHS 1992)

Community hospital beds per 1,000 resident population (U.S.):
1940 = 3.2; 1950 = 3.3; 1960 = 3.6; 1970 = 4.3; 1980 = 4.5; 1989 = 3.8.

Health maintenance organizations (all plans, U.S.):
1976 = 174; 1980 = 235; 1985 = 478; 1986 = 623; 1987 = 647; 1989 = 604; 1990 = 572; 1991 = 553.

Nursing home beds per 1,000 resident population 85 years of age and over (U.S.):
1976 = 681.4; 1982 = 603.0; 1986 = 582.2.

Inpatient and residential treatment beds in mental health organizations per 100,000 civilian population (U.S.):
1970 = 263.6; 1976 = 160.3; 1980 = 124.3; 1988 = 111.5.

Financing: Sources of payment (Levit and Cowan 1991)

Percentage distribution of selected expenditures for health services and supplies (U.S.):

	1965	*1975*	*1980*	*1985*	*1990*
Public					
Federal government	9%	17%	18%	17%	18%
State & local government	12	14	14	15	15
Private					
Private business	17	23	27	28	29
Household (individual)	61	44	38	37	35

Continued

Appendix 7.1   Continued

Characteristics of the Population

Enabling: Regular source of care (Cornelius, Beauregard, and Cohen 1991)

Percentage distribution of regular source of care by race, income (1987):

	Race			Income	
	White	*Black*	*Hispanic*	*High*	*Poor*
None	17.0%	22.9%	27.9%	16.5%	24.0%
Those with location					
Doctor's office	89.5%	69.6%	73.7%	89.5%	73.6%
Hospital OPD, ER	4.4	15.8	9.9	4.4	11.1
Other clinic	6.1	14.5	16.4	6.2	15.3

Enabling: Insurance coverage (Friedman 1991; Ries 1991)

Number of uninsured (est.): 31–37 million; number of underinsured (est.): 48 million.

Percentage of uninsured by race, income (under 65, 1989):

	Race			Income	
	White	*Black*	*Other*	*Nonpoor*	*Poor*
Percent uninsured	12.8%	20.2%	19.7%	10.3%	32.5%

Percentage of poor covered by Medicaid (1989): 40%.

Actual Access

Utilization

Type of use: Use of selected services (NCHS 1992)

Percentage having had procedure or contact by race/ethnicity:

	Race/Ethnicity			
	White	*Black*	*Hispanic*	*Native American*
Began prenatal care, 1st trimester (1989)	78.9%	60.0%	59.5%	57.9%
Vaccinations, children 1–4 (1985)				
— Measles	63.6	48.8	—	—
— Rubella	61.6	47.7	—	—
— DTP	68.7	48.7	—	—
— Polio	58.9	40.1	—	—
— Mumps	61.8	47.0	—	—
Saw dentist, past year (1989)	60.0	44.0	—	—

Continued

Appendix 7.1   Continued

Purpose of use: Use of services relative to need (NCHS 1992)

Physician visits relative to need by race, income (1990):

	Race		Income	
	White	*Black*	*≥$50,000*	*<$14,000*
Need				
Percentage in fair or poor health	8.1%	15.1%	4.0%	18.6%
Percentage with limitation in usual activity due to chronic conditions	12.8	15.5	8.4	22.9
Use				
Percentage saw doctor, past year	78.7	77.5	81.7	77.3
Mean doctor visits, past year	5.6	5.1	5.6	6.3

Satisfaction

General: Public opinion (Blendon and Taylor 1989)

Public's overall view of health care systems (1988):

	U.S.	*Canada*	*U.K.*
— On the whole the health care system works pretty well, and only minor changes are necessary to make it better.	10%	56%	27%
— There are some good things in our health care system, but fundamental changes are needed to make it work better.	60	38	52
— Our health care system has so much wrong with it that we need to completely rebuild it.	29	5	17
— Not sure.	1	1	4

Visit-specific: Patient opinion (Blendon and Taylor 1989)

Patients' satisfaction with medical care (1988):

— Hospitalization: very satisfied.	57%	71%	67%
— Visit to physician: very satisfied.	54%	73%	63%

Appendix 7.2 Criteria for Evaluating Universal Health Insurance Proposals in Terms of the Goal of Equity of Access to Medical Care

Criteria of Equity for Universal Health Insurance Proposals	*Selected Universal Health Insurance Proposals*		
	Government-sponsored, Single-Payer (NHP)	*Employer-Based (PCP)*	*Private Market–Based (CCHP)*
Freedom of Choice			
Minimize constraints on consumer choice of providers.	*Maintain* current care options.	*Encourage* managed care (HMO, PPO, etc.) options.	*Require* managed care (HMO, PPO, etc.) options.
Similar Treatment			
Plan			
Provide universal coverage.	Cover everyone under NHP.	*Private*: Mandate employers cover all employees.	*Private*: Mandate employers cover full-time employees.
	Create public administration of NHP in each state. Phase out all current private and public payers.	*Public*: Create Medicare-like federal program for others. Limit role of Medicaid.	*Public*: Create public sponsors in each state for others. No initial change, Medicaid/Medicare.
Use community rating.	Eliminate private insurance, negotiate budgets, fees.	Reform insurance market; require community rating.	Compensate high-risk plans; maintain experience rating.
Patient			
Use progressive methods to determine consumer contributions.	*Short-run*: Current payers pay into NHP. *Long-run*: Implement payroll, income, or other other progressive tax.	*Private*: Employee pays maximum of 20% of premium.	*Private*: Employer pays maximum of 80% of cost + 8% payroll tax of first $22,500 of salary of employees not covered.

Limit or cap consumer out-of-pocket costs.	No consumer cost-sharing.	*Public:* Enrollee pays maximum of 20% of premium. At poverty level—pay nothing. Up to twice poverty level—sliding scale. Others—full cost. *% max:* 3% of income. *$ max:* $3,000.	*Public: Public sponsor* pays maximum of 80% of cost. At poverty level—cover premium. At 1.5 times poverty level—sliding scale. Others—8% income tax. *max:* 100% of annual premium.
Provider			
Use same reimbursement rates for all payers.	Rates set by *one* payer (NHP).	*Private:* No restrictions. *Public:* Medicare rules.	Rates vary by competing plans.
Limit or cap provider reimbursement.	Global budgets, fees negotiated with NHP.	*Private:* Encourage. *Public:* Require.	Rates negotiated by competing plans.
Decent Basic Minimum			
Cover core benefits: — Primary care — Acute care — Long-term care	*Needed* benefits: Include all services deemed "medically necessary."	*Comprehensive* benefits: Include emphasis on preventive and long-term care.	*Basic* benefits: Include those in HMO Act, with restrictions.
Need, Cost-Effectiveness			
Assign priorities to benefits, based on outcomes: — Primary prevention — Secondary prevention — Tertiary prevention	Establish boards to evaluate necessary and effective services.	Encourage outcomes and effectiveness research; *encourage* "cost-benefit" conscious ("prudent") consumer purchasing.	Encourage outcomes-management research; *require* "cost-quality" conscious employer and consumer choices.
Reform malpractice laws.	—	Study alternatives.	—

Chapter 8

Integrating Health Services Research and Policy Analysis

Health services researchers are routinely involved in producing information used in public policy debates. To further both the producers' and the users' understanding of this research, this chapter examines the relationship between health services research and policy analysis. The first section provides a brief overview of what policy analysts do and why. The objectives of policy analysis are discussed in the context of alternative models of policymaking. Different types of analysis are related to stages of the policymaking process. Next, the role of health services research in policy analysis is explored. Aspects of effectiveness, efficiency, and equity research are related to the policy-analytic tasks of defining the policy problem of interest, identifying and evaluating alternative solutions, and describing and assessing the consequences of specific policy actions. Finally, the limitations of health services research as a resource for policy analysis are reviewed.

Concepts and Methods in Policy Analysis

Objectives of policy analysis

There are two broad objectives of policy analysis: (1) the production of information relevant to policymaking, and (2) the development of reasonable arguments translating the information into recommendations for governmental action (Dunn 1981).[1] The first objective involves conducting or interpreting analyses of individual, institutional, or system behavior related to a given policy question. The findings become the information used to develop an argument supporting a specific policy recommendation. Policy recommendations address the questions policymakers face in determining the need for and direction of government action. Such questions may include the following: (1) what is the problem or opportunity that requires action; (2) what alternatives are likely to resolve the problem or realize the opportunity; and (3) what is the probable or actual success of policies in addressing these issues?

Policymaking may be characterized in general terms as a series of choices about the objectives of government and the means to achieve them. This characterization focuses on decision making and points to the need for both positive (factual) and normative (value-oriented) information.

Positive information is needed, for example, to describe and explain social conditions (the increase in the number of uninsured), the potential consequences of different alternatives being considered to address a problem (the projected number of those without coverage under universal health insurance options), or the actual consequences of existing or past policies (the extent of coverage under existing state-level universal health insurance schemes). The type of question being addressed is factual: does something exist?

Normative information, on the other hand, is needed to determine the desirability of existing conditions, or the worth or value of the consequences produced by a proposed or past action. For example, after providing factual information about the populations that would be covered under various universal health insurance proposals, the analyst may normatively evaluate the proposals according to their potential for achieving a particular equity objective (utilization based on need). The goal of normative analysis is to determine the desirability of current and future conditions. Such information is often a topic of dispute since competing sets of values lead to different interpretations of factual information.

The dual objectives of policy analysis—to conduct relevant analysis and to develop recommendations based on reasonable arguments— suggest criteria for judging policy analysis: relevance, validity, and reasonableness. Relevance refers to the extent to which the normative or factual information the analyst produces is directly linked to policy questions and is timely. Does the information respond to the specific and detailed questions that arise over a bill before Congress or a policy proposal in the governor's office? Its focus must incorporate the specifications of existing programs, proposals, and time frames.

The information that is produced must be valid. Validity in policy analysis refers to the accuracy of information in answering policy questions—that is, identifying the causes of a problem, examining the appropriate set of feasible alternatives, or determining the actual consequences of policy options including the unintended consequences. The more a study fails to meet the above requirements, the less valid it may be deemed to be.

The importance of reasonableness in policy analysis arises from the recognition that the same facts (data showing that health care costs and the number of uninsured are rising) often lead policy stakeholders (interest groups) to conflicting definitions of policy problems or solutions (reforms in health care financing are, or are not, needed). Disagreement over policy claims often focuses on the basic assumptions—such as about human or institutional behavior or the role of government in society—that are often made in translating the data into a claim. In this important sense, all policy claims are subjective. Given the subjective nature of analysis, a primary test of good analysis is whether a given interpretation stands up to critical examination of both its underlying assumptions and its logical structure (Bobrow and Dryzek 1987). Thus, an analysis can be deemed reasonable based on the criterion of completeness. Does it possess policy-relevant information and all the required elements for understanding its logical structure and assumptions?

Dunn (1981) has specified the five components of a complete, reasoned argument:

1. policy-relevant information leading to a recommendation in which the analyst expresses a degree of confidence;
2. warrants to support the recommendation;
3. backing to support further the warrants and recommendation;
4. any special qualifiers to the recommendation; and
5. consideration of possible rebuttals to the argument.

A recommendation that the federal government invest in health maintenance organizations illustrates the nature of each component. The basis of the argument is information that HMOs are more efficient than traditional group or solo practices. A warrant explains why this information leads to the recommendation. In this case, the warrant might refer to the impact of health care costs on the federal budget or to the prospect of the Medicare system becoming insolvent. Further assumptions, arguments, or principles for the recommendation may be needed. Such backing for the HMO investment might include evidence that other cost-control strategies are less effective or have disadvantages compared to the HMO alternative. In the rebuttal, the analyst considers the information, reasons, or assumptions, under which the original claim would be false. The rebuttal in the HMO case might challenge the health care cost impact on the budget, the projected insolvency of

Medicare, or the efficiency claim of HMO supporters. There are two other possible tenets of a rebuttal. First, the policy is not implementable. Second, the strategy has unintended consequences (i.e., on the quality of care).

It should be noted that there are additional uses for policy analysis besides serving as the basis for decision making. For example, analyses may be conducted to reinforce or change policymakers' views about the pros and cons of a policy. The analysis may be conducted to bolster a preconceived position or convince others to change theirs. Another use is predicting the potential for conflict over future decisions. Here, the key is predicting what the relevant decision makers will perceive as the pros and cons of a policy recommendation. Analysis may also be useful in testing and modifying existing theories and methods used in research and analysis. A policy analysis may not have direct influence on current decision making, but it may lead to future efforts that are influential (Nagel 1988).

Models of policymaking

A number of different models of how policy decisions *are* or *should be* made in public and private organizations exist, each with different implications for the role and type of policy analysis that is possible or appropriate. These include the rational-comprehensive, satisficing, mixed-scanning, and political models.

The *rational-comprehensive* model of decision making, which dates back to the philosophical writings of John Dewey (1910) and other American pragmatists, depicts the policymaking process as a series of logical, well-defined stages (see Table 8.1):

1. defining the problem;
2. identifying alternatives with the potential to solve the problem;
3. evaluating and selecting an alternative that best meets the goals;
4. describing the consequences of the selected alternative; and
5. evaluating and modifying the alternative in light of its consequences.

This model idealizes the policymaker as an objective, well-informed individual whose goal is to select policies that maximize community welfare. The model suggests a chronological sequence of analyses to resolve problems in a logical and orderly manner. In its extreme, this model implies a major role for comprehensive policy analysis. The analysis must consider all possible definitions of a problem, express policy goals clearly and specifically, include a thorough examination of all potential alternatives in developing a resolution, and evaluate their possible consequences based on the performance of related actions.

Recognizing that information for policy analysis is both limited and costly to obtain leads to the realization that in many instances decisions must be made under conditions of uncertainty. This limitation leads to the *incremental view* (also referred to as the *satisficing* model) of policymaking, which is probably more descriptive of the actual policymaking process than the rational-comprehensive model (Lindblom 1959; Simon 1982). In the satisficing model, the goal is more to alleviate shortcomings in current policy than to find the best possible course of action. Whereas the rational-comprehensive model looks for the best alternative course of action from many alternatives, the satisficing model chooses the first alternative that is deemed an acceptable (or satisficing) one. Analyses of different questions are done in an iterative rather than sequential manner, with policymakers continuously reformulating problems and potential solutions. The role of policy analysis is much more limited than in the rational-comprehensive model. The emphasis is on supplying feedback as policy moves incrementally toward an optimal solution.

The *mixed-scanning model* (Etzioni 1967) proposes that strategic (long-term) decisions that set basic policy directions be based on rational-comprehensive analysis but that operational (short-term) choices, which

Table 8.1 Stages of Policymaking, Relevant Information, and Type of Research

Stages of Policymaking	*Relevant Information*	*Type of Research*
1. Defining problems	Scope, severity, causes, importance of the problem	Conceptual analyses and descriptive studies of the problems and causes
2. Identifying alternatives	Forecasts of likely consequences of alternatives	Conceptual and empirical projections of the consequences of alternatives
3. Evaluating alternatives	Normative evaluations prior to action	Conceptual applications of frameworks for normative evaluation of alternatives
4. Describing consequences	Process and impact of policies and programs	Descriptive studies of program and policy effects
5. Evaluating consequences	Normative evaluations subsequent to action	Normative studies of program and policy effects

deal more with implementing broad strategies, be based on satisficing (or incremental) analysis.

These three models, rational-comprehensive, satisficing, and mixed-scanning, are all variants on the rational approach to policymaking. They all imply a substantial decision making role for policy analysis. None, however, principally takes into account the political nature of the process.

In contrast to these three rational models of policy analysis, the *political model* emphasizes the political context for policymaking with its multiplicity of goals, values, and interests that influence policy (Stone 1988). It challenges the assumption that policymakers are motivated solely to provide rational solutions to social problems and that institutions are structured to facilitate objective analysis of problems and alternatives (Jones 1976). This model describes the policy process more in terms of conflict resolution and consensus building. Problems and solutions addressed in the policy process reflect the individual goals of conflicting interest groups rather than the products of objective analysis. Outcomes of the policy process depend more on the ability of these affected groups to organize and participate in the political process than on the extent to which some policy achieves a given performance objective.

The symbolic analogy of the garbage can is used to depict the political model's more irrational and nonsystematic approach to decision making (March and Olsen 1976). The mix of garbage in the can depends on what garbage is being produced at the moment, the number of cans available, and the speed with which garbage is collected and removed from the scene. It suggests a relatively minor role for policy analysis aimed primarily at predicting the potential conflicts among stakeholders participating in the decision-making process.

Despite the limitations of the rational model and its variants as a description of the policy process, it does clearly illuminate the types of research and relevant information required for rational decision making. It is therefore adopted here as a basis for clarifying the role of health services research in policy analysis, with the following qualifications.

The stages specified in the rational model do not simply imply a strategy of carrying out the analysis relevant to a stage, completing that stage, moving to the next stage, and so forth. This would be inappropriate for a number of reasons. As discussed previously, the limits of information and the extent to which the environment is politicized lead to a process that is more iterative than sequential. Also, it is important to consider the implications of each stage in advance of actually carrying it out, for example, taking into account the possible problems of implementation (Stage 4) when initially evaluating alternatives (Stage 3) (Hogwood and Gunn 1984). In situations where the analysis, or the options suggested for a given stage, may have already been precluded by prior decisions, such an analysis would obviously be irrelevant. The limits of information and the political nature of the process in a given context must also be considered in determining the type of analysis appropriate to a given question.

In the remainder of this chapter the types of analysis that are suggested by each stage of the rational model are discussed. The analyses should not be viewed as a substitute for the judgment, insight, and creativity of the policymaker. It is suggested, however, that more-systematic analysis at different stages of the policy process will enhance policymakers' rational decision making.

Policymaking and policy analysis

The policy analyst must select from a variety of research frameworks and methods in addressing policy questions. The appropriateness of a particular approach depends on the kind of question being asked, which, in turn, depends on the stage of the policy process. This section describes the goals and types of analysis appropriate to each stage. Table 8.1 lists the types of policy decisions associated with the five stages of the rational model, the information needed to inform the policymaker at each stage, and the various types of research and analysis that are relevant.

Defining problems

The general objective of Stage 1, defining problems, is to identify a failure of the current system to meet some defined performance goal. Three types of information are relevant at this stage: normative arguments assessing the importance of various policy objectives (effectiveness, efficiency, and equity); descriptive information relating prevailing policy conditions to a more-ideal mix of objectives or a higher level of each; and conceptual and empirical analyses explaining the causes of existing conditions and suggesting possible solutions. The first task is to clarify the norms for judging a situation problematic. This task is necessitated by the fact that a problem exists only when there is a discrepancy between what ought to be and what is. The task is difficult because many times there is general concern about a situation but no agreement on a precise standard to use in defining it as a problem.

To clarify policy norms, one can conduct population surveys or review reports from public hearings or focus groups specifying common views on objectives and concerns. One can ask the relevant policymaking body, or rely on some kind of observational analysis of past decisions, legislation, testimony, or other written material to infer what the norms might be (Nagel 1988). Sometimes expert panels can provide a standard, i.e., the Agency for Health Care Policy and Research clinical guidelines process described in Chapter 3 offers a standard for judging problems with Medicare coverage policy. There are even rare occasions when government officials have defined in specific terms a standard of "what ought to be," such as the Hill-Burton standard for the ratio of hospital beds to population.

The second task is to describe what initially are usually vague and often conflicting perceptions of an undesirable situation in more precise and systematic terms. The objective is to define the scope and magnitude of the problem in terms of affected individuals or institutions. For example, to address concerns about the high cost of medical care services, the analyst might try to locate data showing how costs are growing, how the growth in medical service cost relates to other economic indicators such as wages or price inflation, and how the cost burden on third-party payers and patients is distributed.

The third task is to conceptualize the problem, classifying it and explaining the relationships between its different dimensions. Theoretical and empirical models or frames of reference are necessary to classify a problem. For example, people may disagree about the kind of problem represented by rapidly rising health care costs, uneven distribution of physicians, and surplus hospital beds. Studies of effects of health insurance coverage on hospital use and costs, research on factors affecting physicians' choices of practice locations, and inquiries about determinants of hospital capital expenditures are illustrations of the types of research likely to help define and classify the problem. Successful completion of these three Stage 1 tasks leads to suggested solutions through understanding the dimensions of the problem and its probable causes.

Identifying alternatives

At Stage 2, the analyst seeks to select policy alternatives that have the potential to correct, compensate for, or counteract the causes of the problem. The projected consequences of an alternative are the relevant information for Stage 2 analysis. Statistical models and simulation techniques may aid the analyst in generating quantitative projections of policy consequences. For example, the Physician Payment Review Commission compared baseline projections of physician payments under the Medicare RBRVS fee schedule (prior to its actual implementation) with payments under the customary, prevailing, and reasonable charge methodology (Colby 1992). It is perhaps more common to rely on theoretical reasoning (inductive or deductive) to generate estimates of projected consequences, an approach illustrated in Chapter 4 relative to the debate about whether market incentives are better than government regulations for generating efficient allocation of scarce resources. Economic theory is often used to suggest that market incentives will lead to allocative efficiency. Such projections are based upon deductive reasoning from assumptions about the behavioral responses of providers and consumers to certain market conditions.

Evaluating alternatives

The projected consequences of policy alternatives are evaluated in terms of defined policy goals or objectives at Stage 3. Analytical tasks are: identifying the mix of goals that are to be used to evaluate different alternatives, translating them into criteria (quantitative or qualitative) that capture the important dimensions of each goal, and specifying the effects of alternatives in terms of those criteria (Weimer and Vining 1989). For example, to evaluate alternative proposals for emergency transportation services, the analyst may define the average rush-hour delay for vehicles as the criterion related to the goal of improving access to urban trauma centers. Changes in the cost of private ambulances may be another criterion derived from the goal of economic efficiency. The analyst must then apply these criteria to policy alternatives and clarify the trade-offs between the goals suggested by each alternative.

A practical difficulty arises when the analyst combines multiple goals to develop an overall assessment of alternatives. Various decision models or optimum-choice frameworks are available to assist the analyst with this problem. Some of the more rigorous include: cost-benefit analysis, multiattribute utility analysis, threshold analysis, optimum-mix analysis, and multigoal analysis (McKenna 1980; Nagel 1988; Stokey and Zeckhauser 1978). Unfortunately, the application of these models requires quantitative data and a level of precision that is often not available to policy analysts.

Describing consequences

The analytic objective of Stage 4 is twofold: to determine the degree to which a policy or program was implemented as intended and to measure both anticipated and unanticipated effects. Monitoring implementation asks if certain standards are being followed or if the policy or program reflects appropriate use of resources. Specific indicators often used in monitoring include measures of inputs (personnel, facilities, equipment, supplies); processes (administrative, organizational, clinical, behavioral, political, attitudinal); outputs (goods and services provided); and effects (health status of target groups). In measuring effects, the analyst attempts to determine whether a policy has brought about change in, for example, the behavior, attitudes, or health status of targeted individuals, groups, organizations, or communities. Methods for determining effects range from social systems accounting—in which the analyst monitors overall changes in health or other social status indicators (such as infant mortality rates) over time and attempts to relate the changes logically to policy in general—to experimental and quasi-experimental evaluations of specific programs (such as prenatal care access interventions) designed explicitly to isolate the effects of the programs from other factors (overall downward trends in infant mortality) (Shortell and Richardson 1978).

Evaluating consequences

At Stage 5 of policymaking, evaluating consequences, policymakers may use performance information in deciding whether to continue, modify, or terminate existing policies, or to redefine the original problem. To assess performance analytically, the consequences of a policy are evaluated normatively in light of designated goals and criteria. The menu of analytic approaches described for Stage 3 of the policy process (evaluating alternatives) is also relevant to Stage 5, but the focus of Stage 5 is on evaluating *actual* rather than *potential* consequences. To evaluate performance, the analyst must define the goals for policy, transform them into criteria that can be used in evaluation, and apply them to the consequences of a policy or program. As discussed earlier, the identification and use of norms in policy analysis is plagued with difficulties. Policymakers may not be able to decide on the appropriate goals in a particular context, they almost never decide on the appropriate trade-offs between pairs of these goals, and they may have implicit goals (hidden agendas) that they are unwilling to make explicit. Alternative approaches to resolving such conflicts were listed earlier in the section on decision models.

The Role of Health Services Research in Policy Analysis

As described in the previous chapters, health services research seeks to clarify the goals of the health care system in terms of the equity, effectiveness, and efficiency of service delivery. Criteria, methods, and data sources have been developed for evaluating the degree to which performance goals in these areas are being realized and for identifying what alternatives might assist in improving the performance of the system. The discussion that follows relates this research to policy analysis by describing the usefulness of health services research in defining policy problems, identifying and evaluating alternatives, and describing and evaluating the consequences of policy decisions.

Defining problems

As mentioned previously, policy goals must be made clear as a basis for defining problems requiring government action. There are two fundamentally different tasks involved. One is to determine what the goals *ought to be*. This is largely a values question that is subject to differing views of the nature of medical care and the role of the health care system. The second is to *suggest measures and techniques* for clarifying goals and relating them to policy choices about the existence of problems and the selection of solutions. The latter task is addressed by the concepts and methods used in health services research that help to clarify and operationalize the standards of effectiveness, efficiency, and equity for use in policy analysis.

Effectiveness

As indicated in Chapter 2, the health services research literature suggests two possible ways of defining the goal of effectiveness in policy analysis, one focusing broadly on benefits to the population, and the other focusing more narrowly on benefits to the individual patient (Figure 2.1). From the population perspective, effectiveness is defined as the proportion of the population with a problem who are benefited by treatment. It is measured by the product of the percentage of problems brought to medical care, the percentage prescribed treatment, the rate of patient compliance with that treatment, and the efficacy of the treatment provided (Table 2.2). Policy analysis aimed at improving effectiveness defined and measured in this way could compare medical care with other population-oriented strategies for improving the quality and quantity of life. The benefits achieved by addressing inadequate housing, smoking, and drug abuse, and by improving job skills, might be contrasted with those resulting from a more effective system of medical care delivery. Explicit analyses of the health effects of patient behavior and environmental conditions as well as the quality of medical care are relevant in this perspective.

An alternative definition of effectiveness focuses more narrowly on the benefits achieved by patients receiving medical care under conditions of actual practice. Analyses using this definition have a traditional clinical perspective. The evaluation standard might be stated in terms of actual benefits in medical practice compared to maximum achievable benefits (efficacy). This measure is relevant when the emphasis is on improving the performance of medical care providers as opposed to the medical care system as a whole (see Table 2.3).

Efficiency

The policy goal of efficiency in medical care may also be approached in two ways: encouraging the right mix of medical care services to maximize social welfare (allocative efficiency), or encouraging the right mix of medical inputs and production methods to maximize productivity (production efficiency). Criteria for analysis in both cases include production and cost standards deduced from microeconomic theory and measures derived from applying the cost-effectiveness or cost-benefit frameworks.

The microeconomic model of the medical care provider shows the relationship between different levels and mixes of inputs, input prices, and technology to minimize the cost of services. It can be used in policy analysis when the concern is with the production of a specific service or mix of services. For example, each setting for health care—such as a medical practice, hospital, or nursing home—uses a particular combination of health personnel, supported by other inputs, to produce services. The microeconomic model suggests criteria that can be used to identify empirically the most-efficient combination of personnel to support a particular level of medical service.

The cost-effectiveness framework, on the other hand, may be used when the concern is with comparing the relative efficiency of policies or programs that try to achieve the same objective through alternative methods of production. A cost-effectiveness ratio (e.g., cost per medical encounter, per case found, or per quality-adjusted life-year) is computed and compared among the alternatives. It is important to note that production efficiency also requires that services be effective. Efficiency analysis must be preceded by the technical appraisal of clinical or population-based effectiveness.

The broader goal of allocative efficiency is assessed using the cost-benefit framework. The analyst calculates and compares the costs and benefits of a policy, program, or service to determine if it adds to social welfare. All relevant social costs and benefits must be identified and measured in dollars, if possible, so that comparisons (costs versus benefits) can be made across all possible actions. Future costs and benefits must be discounted to reflect their present value. Subtracting costs from benefits yields net benefits, the criterion indicating increased social welfare. Allocative inefficiencies are indicated when the aggregate costs of a policy or program exceed its aggregate benefits.

Equity

As discussed in Chapter 6, equity goals derive from ethical principles of distributive justice regarding the fair distribution of the benefits and burdens of medical care (Figure 6.1). While there continues to be debate about which norms should serve as the basis for defining equity in medical care delivery, specific distributional goals and criteria can be derived that embody aspects of a number of alternative theories of distributive justice (Table 6.1). Each can, in turn, be translated into empirical indicators of access to care as explained in Chapter 6 to evaluate the extent to which equity has been achieved. Equity-of-access indicators include the characteristics of the delivery system (the availability and distribution of services), the characteristics of the population (ethnicity, gender, insurance coverage, regular source of care), the use of services, and satisfaction with services (Table 6.2). Equity-of-access goals may be evaluated at the system, institutional, or community level by applying these indicators (Table 6.3).

Identifying and evaluating alternatives

In addition to identifying and clarifying problems, health services research is helpful to policymakers in determining desirable strategies for solving problems. Theoretical models may be adopted as the "rational" foundation for new proposals. In other instances, both theory and empirical studies may be applied to depicting the potential success of a strategy.

Effectiveness

The structure-process-outcomes framework developed by Donabedian (1966) as the conceptual guide for effectiveness research is useful in the policy-analytic task of a priori identification and evaluation of policy or program alternatives. This framework may be applied at the population level, with medical care viewed as one of the inputs contributing to the health of the population, to evaluate what can be done to improve the effectiveness of medical care through manipulation of system variables. It can also be used as the basis for analysis at the clinical level, to evaluate what can be done to improve clinical practice.

The framework suggests the kind of data needed to identify possible solutions to an effectiveness problem. Evidence linking the elements of the framework to outcomes suggests targets for interventions. For example, in clarifying a policymaker's concern about the quality of care in nursing homes, the structure-process-outcomes framework suggests that the quality of nursing home care is influenced by structural factors such as the quantity of staff and their qualifications. Quality, in turn, has an influence on outcomes including mortality, morbidity, functional status, and client satisfaction. The framework indicates the structure and process factors that should be manipulated by policy alternatives designed to improve the effectiveness of care.

Efficiency

Research concerned with allocative and production efficiency informs policymakers about what alternatives tend to result in the provision of effective services that are relatively inexpensive to deliver. Numerous empirical studies, for example, document that physicians and hospitals generally could use nonphysician inputs more efficiently (Reinhardt 1975; Smith, Miller, and Golladay 1972), that HMO patients' use of hospitals is much less than fee-for-service patients' with no corresponding reduction in the effectiveness of care (Luft 1981), and that cost sharing results in lower use and cost of medical care with little or no decline in health status for the average patient (Manning et al. 1987). Researchers are attempting to provide better information on the efficiency of a variety of specific medical care services aimed at common medical problems and the resources, organizational arrangements, and financing mechanisms involved in their provision.

Solutions to efficiency problems may also be identified and evaluated through analysis of medical care market conditions (see Chapter 4). Microeconomic theory suggests market conditions that lead to inefficiencies in production or allocation if not corrected. Many of these conditions have been shown to be present in medical care markets. For example, the uncertain consequences of some types of medical care make it difficult for patients to judge what is in their best interest. The external benefits and costs of some types of medical care (for example, immunization to prevent infectious disease, which benefits populations as well as individuals) may not be appropriately valued by private markets, leading to inefficient allocation. The gap in knowledge between patients and providers leaves patients vulnerable to inappropriate care or care they would not choose for themselves if they were well informed. Documenting the presence of such adverse conditions is another method used by analysts to identify government interventions designed to improve efficiency.

It should be noted that applying the competitive economic model to enhance efficiency in health care assumes that maximizing satisfaction of consumer preferences is an appropriate policy goal. This is a value judgment that should be clearly stated when applying the model. An alternative model that emphasizes maximizing the population's health status (or meeting medical care needs) is a substitute for consumer satisfaction in efficiency analysis. Both models are briefly discussed in Chapters 2 and 4. Criteria for judging the determinants of allocative efficiency in the needs-based model are not as well developed as in the competitive economic model.

Equity

Empirical analyses of the relative importance of various factors presumed to influence whether or not people receive care, and how satisfied they are, point to possible points of intervention for health policy to enhance equity of access. Access indicators discussed earlier may be used to identify potential solutions to an equity problem through examining the correlation of these indicators with *actual* access measures—utilization and satisfaction. Those factors that most directly influence access to needed services (such as insurance coverage or a regular source of medical care) then become the focus of the design and implementation of programs and services to enhance access.

Like efficiency analysis, access research assumes that services are effective, that is, that gaining access to care could make a difference in improving people's health. Access indicators incorporating norms regarding those conditions that medical care can help to ameliorate (sentinel events, avoidable hospitalizations, or ambulatory care–sensitive conditions) embody both the equity *and* effectiveness criteria (Weissman, Gatsonis, and Epstein 1992).

Describing and evaluating consequences

Effectiveness

Effectiveness research supplies the conceptual framework, methods, and evidence that are used by policy analysts to describe and evaluate specific policy strategies. Research linking structural factors—the quantity and efficacy of medical inputs—to health outcomes can be conducted to assess the impact of a particular intervention on desired policy outcomes. In the same way, studies on the effects of process—the quantity, quality, and appropriateness of services delivered—on medical outcomes guide us in evaluating the success of options to change the process of medical care delivery. Analysts use this information in measuring the consequences (higher patient survival rates) of any given solution (regional centers for open-heart surgery), which can then be related to desired policy objectives (to improve the effectiveness of medical services).

Efficiency

The concepts, definitions, and methods health economists have developed to examine the allocative and production efficiency of medical care are important resources for describing and assessing the consequences of policy actions. There are numerous studies of production efficiency, as outlined in Chapter 5, to guide evaluations of the organization and production of medical services. The RAND Health Insurance Experiment discussed in prior chapters is a good example of this kind of research carried out with a rigorous, large-scale, experimental design. Findings indicated the costs and effects of alternative insurance strategies ranging from first-dollar coverage to catastrophic plans. Estimates were made of the excess spending that occurred under first-dollar coverage, given the low marginal value of the added medical care services consumed. Studies of the efficiency of prepaid group practice are another important example. Many well-conducted cost-effectiveness studies (Chapter 5) that provide useful information on the relative efficiency of alternative services and technologies are also available.

Equity

Both analytic research and evaluative research are relevant to the task of describing and evaluating the consequences of health policy on access. Analytic research suggests causes of access problems that are likely to be altered by private or government interventions. Empirical measurement of the effects of specific factors (e.g., social support available to high-risk mothers) form the primary basis for evaluating the equity consequences (e.g., prenatal care utilization rates) of alternative policy options (e.g., case management services). Evaluative research on access (reviewed in Chapter 6) is useful in actually informing policy analysts of the success of *specific* programs or policies to enhance access.

Difficulties in linking health services research to policy

To the extent that the conceptual theories and empirical studies from effectiveness, efficiency, and equity research are not well developed or clear, the research is limited as a source of knowledge for policy analysis. The prior sections reviewed the potential contributions of health services research to policy analysis, while the discussion that follows highlights some of the limitations.

Effectiveness

No policy or professional consensus exists on whether the population or clinical perspective is more appropriate for defining effectiveness in medical care delivery. The clinical perspective leaves out important factors that contribute to the health of the population. The population perspective requires that health policy address factors beyond the medical care system (e.g., housing and jobs). As indicated in Chapter 2, the clinical perspective has become more prominent of late, with the emphasis on research evaluating the outcomes of specific clinical practices. Related to the debate over perspectives is the question of how health is to be defined. From the population perspective, community health indicators are important. From the clinical perspective, individual patient health status and satisfaction are emphasized.

The lack of standards for effective medical practice is a critical weakness in applying effectiveness analysis at the clinical and population levels. Only rough estimates can be made in addressing questions concerning the relationships between structure and outcomes, and between processes and outcomes of care. Studies of variations in practice indicate that there is an extremely wide range of acceptable practice patterns (Chassin, Brook, and Park 1986; Eisenberg and Nicklin 1981; Roos 1984; Schroeder, Kenders, and Cooper 1973; Wennberg and Gittelsohn 1982). However, notwithstanding the recent efforts by the federal government to invest in this type of research, we are unable to determine precisely how much of the variation can be attributed to the provision of ineffective services.

Efficiency

Efficiency research provides useful but limited information on the optimal allocation of resources and production methods. We are only beginning to understand the effect of medical care and other investments on health and well-being for many important medical services. Without this information, the social value of resource-allocation decisions cannot be determined with precision. The relative efficiency of different organizational models and resource mixes for producing medical care are not clear despite the extensive research in some areas, for example, comparing HMO and fee-for-service models of physician care and hospital inpatient versus outpatient settings for the provision of various procedures and services. A conceptual difficulty when applying allocative efficiency criteria for evaluating policy alternatives is that the distributional consequences of alternatives (some win and some lose as a result) cannot be assessed. We can use Pareto optimum criteria that the beneficiaries compensate the payers (Chapter 4), but this may not be ethically acceptable if there are no mechanisms for ensuring that winners compensate losers.

Equity

The focus of research on equity would be enhanced if there were greater theoretical and political consensus on what equity means. Chapter 6 proposes a multidimensional goal that incorporates the elements of alternative theories of distributive justice. Some of the dimensions have the potential for conflict, making it difficult to apply the criteria in policy analysis. Equity research also shares with effectiveness and efficiency research a lack of analytic precision. The causal relationships between *actual* access and *potential* access indicators have not been thoroughly and uniformly documented. More research is also needed on indicators that embody both the effectiveness and equity criteria, that is, indicators of access to those services for which medical care *can* make a difference.

This chapter describes competing models of the policy process and their implications for policy analysis. The rational-comprehensive model is selected as a guide that policy analysts and health services researchers can use to identify the types of research relevant to specific health policy questions. This model identifies the sequential stages of the policymaking process and the information and types of research required to guide decision making at each stage. The stages of the rational-comprehensive model best serve to illuminate the *empirical* bridges between health services research and policy analysis.

Note

1. Our discussion focuses on public policymaking. However, the concepts, terms, and methods presented are generally applicable to the private sector as well.

References

Bobrow, D., and J. Dryzek. 1987. *Policy Analysis by Design*. Pittsburgh: University of Pittsburgh Press.
Chassin, M., R. Brook, and R. Park. 1986. "Variations in the Use of Medical and Surgical Services by the Medicare Population." *New England Journal of Medicine* 314: 285–90.
Colby, D. 1992. "Impact of the Medicare Physician Fee Schedule." *Health Affairs* 11 (3): 216–26.
Dewey, J. 1910. *How We Think*. New York: D.C. Heath and Company.
Donabedian, A. 1966. "Evaluating the Quality of Medical Care." *Milbank Memorial Fund Quarterly* 44: 166–206.
Dunn, W. 1981. *Public Policy Analysis*. Englewood Cliffs, NJ: Prentice-Hall.
Eisenberg, J., and D. Nicklin. 1981. "Use of Diagnostic Services by Physicians in Community Practice." *Medical Care* 19: 297–309.
Etzioni, A. 1967. "Mixed Scanning: A 'Third' Approach to Decision Making." *Public Administration Review* 27: 385–92.
Hogwood, B., and L. Gunn. 1984. *Policy Analysis for the Real World*. New York: Oxford University Press.

Jones, C. 1976. "Why Congress Can't Do Policy Analysis (or Words to That Effect)." *Policy Analysis* 2: 251–64.

Lindblom, C. 1959. "The Science of Muddling Through." *Public Administration Review* 19: 79–88.

Luft, H. 1981. *Health Maintenance Organizations: Dimensions of Performance.* New York: Wiley Interscience.

Manning, W., J. Newhouse, N. Duan, E. Keeler, A. Leibowitz, and S. Marquis. 1987. "Health Insurance and the Demand for Medical Care: Evidence from a Randomized Experiment." *American Economic Review* 77 (3): 251–77.

March, J., and J. Olsen. 1976. *Ambiguity and Choice in Organizations.* Oslo, Norway: Universitetsforlaget.

McKenna, C. 1980. *Quantitative Methods for Public Decision Making.* New York: McGraw-Hill Book Company.

Nagel, S. 1988. *Policy Studies: Integration and Evaluation.* Westport, CT: Greenwood Press.

Reinhardt, U. E. 1975. *Physician Productivity and the Demand for Health Manpower.* Cambridge, MA: Ballinger Publishing Company.

Roos, N. 1984. "Hysterectomy: Variation in Rates across Small Areas and across Physicians' Practices." *American Journal of Public Health* 71: 606–12.

Schroeder, S., K. Kenders, and J. Cooper. 1973. "Use of Laboratory Tests and Pharmaceuticals: Variation among Physicians and Effect of Cost Audit on Subsequent Use." *Journal of the American Medical Association* 225: 969–73.

Shortell, S., and W. Richardson. 1978. *Health Program Evaluation.* St. Louis: C.V. Mosby.

Simon, H. 1982. *Models of Bounded Rationality.* Cambridge, MA: MIT Press.

Smith, K., M. Miller, and F. Golladay. 1972. "An Analysis of the Optimal Use of Inputs in the Production of Medical Services." *Journal of Human Resources* 7: 208–55.

Stokey, E., and R. Zeckhauser. 1978. *A Primer for Policy Analysis.* New York: W. W. Norton & Co.

Stone, D. 1988. *Policy Paradox and Political Reason.* Glenview, IL: Scott, Foresman and Co.

Weimer, D., and A. Vining. 1989. *Policy Analysis: Concepts and Practice.* Englewood Cliffs, NJ: Prentice-Hall.

Weissman, J., C. Gatsonis, and A. Epstein. 1992. "Rates of Avoidable Hospitalization by Insurance Status in Massachusetts and Maryland." *Journal of the American Medical Association* 268: 2388–94.

Wennberg, J., and A. Gittelsohn. 1982. "Variations in Medical Care among Small Areas." *Scientific American* 246: 120–34.

Chapter 9

Applying Health Services
Research to Policy Analysis

This chapter concludes the book with an illustration in which effectiveness, efficiency, and equity research are applied in a prospective evaluation of universal health insurance alternatives. The major provisions of three diverse UHI proposals are described, and their projected consequences are evaluated. The analysis is patterned after analyses that have appeared in the health services research literature at other times when national health reform appeared to be just around the corner.

Somers and Somers (1977, 132) suggested that UHI proposals be evaluated in terms of the goal of ensuring universal access, and they put forth the following goal statement as a guide for their analysis: "universal access, as needed, to personal health services along with adequate personnel and facilities, quality protection, and controlled costs." They argued, based on a critical review of Medicare and Medicaid, that a single, national, uniform program financed primarily with taxes is required to achieve universal access.

Feldstein (1988) used neoclassical economic theory to identify criteria by which UHI proposals should be judged. He suggested an overall goal of achieving a desirable distribution of necessary medical services while allowing the maximum possible degree of consumer choice. By applying economic analysis, he inferred the following desirable provisions for UHI: (1) tax credits and deductions determined on the basis of income to encourage broader insurance coverage; (2) direct in-kind subsidies to those with very low incomes; (3) deductibles and copayments for individuals to achieve cost control, with an upper limit on liability for medical expenses; (4) provider payment provisions that put providers at risk for the cost of care; and (5) progressive public financing designed to have minimal effects on the price of goods and services or the demand for labor.

Brown (1988) systematically evaluated the major dimensions of several UHI proposals that had been introduced in Congress, using seven criteria: inclusiveness of population coverage, comprehensiveness of benefits, equity in financing, efficiency in resource use, planning in the allocation of resources, mechanisms for accountability, and political feasibility. Brown applied each criterion as a continuum, with one end of the continuum the desirable provisions of a UHI plan and the other end the undesirable provisions. For example, inclusiveness of coverage translated into a continuum with segmented programs at the undesirable end and a single universal program at the desirable end. Brown then ranked the coverage provisions of different proposals by their location on each continuum. Overall rankings of UHI proposals were derived by examining the rankings on each criterion.

These approaches define three contrasting conceptual and normative bases for evaluating UHI alternatives. The Somers and Somers analysis focused on the normative goal of equity defined as universal access. Feldstein emphasized economic efficiency defined in terms of consumer satisfaction. Brown identified and applied a number of diverse evaluative criteria to the key components of UHI alternatives (e.g., coverage, benefits, financing). The analytical approach to evaluating UHI proposals presented here extends Brown's approach of evaluating the major provisions of competing proposals to an explicit consideration of the norms of effectiveness, efficiency, and equity.

The analysis begins by describing eight major features of three diverse proposals and locating the proposals on a series of continua reflecting their use of market-minimizing versus market-maximizing strategies. (See Figure 9.1.) As discussed in Chapter 4, market-minimizing strategies tend to favor public provision of medical insurance financed by taxes and administered by national or state agencies. Market-maximizing strategies, on the other hand, rely more on private insurance companies to underwrite benefits, with financing through premiums. This dichotomy was selected to highlight the critical differences that are the focus of UHI policy debate.

The proposals are compared by considering, for each provision, whether their market-minimizing or market-maximizing strategies are most likely to achieve the goals of effectiveness, efficiency, and equity. Empirical and conceptual research is cited to evaluate the consequences of the strategies. When possible, the proposals are ranked on each provision by evaluating the extent to which their proposed strategies would maximize effectiveness, efficiency, and equity.

Figure 9.1 Dimensions for Evaluating Universal Health Insurance Proposals

UHI Proposals Dimensions	NHP *Market- Minimized*	PCP		CCHP *Market- Maximized*
1. Who is covered?	Everyone	← Efficiency Equity	→	Targeted
2. How are they covered?	Mandated, single-payer	← Equity	Efficiency →	Voluntary, competing plans
3. What is the basis for determining coverage?	Need	← Effectiveness Equity	Efficiency →	Demand
4. What is the basis for determining payment methods and prices?	Publicly administered	← Equity	→	Market-determined
5. What is the extent of consumer copayments?	None	← Equity	Effectiveness Efficiency →	Extensive
6. How would it be financed?	Taxes	← Equity	Efficiency →	Premiums to private insurers
7. How would it be administered?	Government	←	→	Multiple private insurers
8. How would costs be controlled?	Spending caps, planning, and technology limits	← Effectiveness Equity	→	Consumer and provider incentives

Note: The words "effectiveness," "efficiency," and "equity" appear along a given continuum according to which proposal or proposals receive the highest rating for the respective norm on that continuum. No word appears for a norm when the highest rating is not clear on that continuum.

Description and Evaluation of the Proposals

The UHI proposals to be reviewed are: the National Health Program, a market-minimizing approach based on a single plan administered by the government (Grumbach et al. 1991; Himmelstein et al. 1989); the Consumer Choice Health Plan, a market-maximizing approach relying on financial incentives and regulated competition to encourage efficiency, effectiveness, and equity (Enthoven and Kronick 1989a, 1989b, 1991); and the Pepper Commission proposal, which balances the two approaches by calling on employers to provide health insurance or pay a payroll tax to fund a government-administered plan and looking to a combination of government regulation and market competition to contain costs (Pepper Commission 1990). While there are a variety of other UHI proposals being touted at both the national and state levels, these three encompass the diverse themes that are represented in the debate. Figure 9.1 locates the proposals on the multidimensional continua, highlighting their market-minimizing and market-maximizing features. Each proposal's strategies for addressing the eight major provisions of UHI are described and evaluated below. (See Appendix 7.2 for a summary of the major features of each plan.)

1. Who is covered?   2. How are they covered?

Description

On the left of Figure 9.1 is the market-minimizing system proposed by the NHP, in which everyone is enrolled in a plan administered by the government or its intermediaries. Insurance companies would be prohibited from selling insurance for services provided under the government plan. On the right of the figure is the market-maximizing CCHP, which mandates employer-sponsored insurance or taxation for business, market-enhancing taxation provisions and insurance regulations, continuation of Medicare and Medicaid, and a voucher system to enable the non-Medicaid and non-Medicare poor to purchase private insurance. The PCP, in the center of the figure, mandates employer-sponsored insurance or an insurance tax by large business, strong financial incentives for employee coverage by small business, and a single national health plan for those outside the labor force.

The NHP guarantees coverage of the entire population, replacing employer-sponsored insurance for health services with one government plan. The other two proposals guarantee coverage in a national plan for certain groups and provide subsidies and tax incentives to others to encourage the voluntary purchase of private insurance. In the PCP, employers with more than 100 employees must provide health insurance coverage for them or pay a payroll tax. Small businesses would be encouraged to cover their employees through incentives and small-group insurance reforms. Nonworkers and the self-employed would be covered by a federally administered public plan that would replace Medicaid. The CCHP is even more targeted and voluntary. Full-time employees would be covered by employers or a publicly sponsored plan. Everyone else would be covered by either a public sponsor, Medicare, or Medicaid. Actual coverage would depend on individual choices in response to tax incentives and how active public sponsors were in marketing their plans.

Evaluation

Effectiveness. Mortality data from countries with a national health system, such as the United Kingdom, suggest that all levels of society benefit from universal coverage. The data show that the use of health services increases for all levels, and that all types of mortality decline over time. However, the gaps in population health measures, between those at the lowest level of society and those at the highest level, either stay the same or increase (Hollingsworth 1981). These findings have two implications. On the one hand, they confirm that universal coverage contributes to the goal of improving the health of the population. On the other hand, they suggest that a more-targeted approach to medical care coverage, one that favors low-income groups, may be needed to close the health status gap between low-income and high-income groups.

This research is ambiguous with respect to the three proposals. The NHP ranks above the other two in terms of its potential for improving the health of the population as a whole, since it mandates universal coverage. However, the PCP and CCHP may be more likely to close the gap between rich and poor by adopting the more-targeted approach of subsidizing the coverage of low-income groups more heavily than others.

Efficiency. Coverage is a demand-side issue and therefore has consequences for the issue of allocative efficiency. In most markets, consumers are able to choose freely whether or not to purchase a product according to what they feel is in their own best interest. When the market is competitive and there are no externalities (negative or positive effects on third parties), this freedom of choice tends to result in allocative efficiency. However, given the nature of health, health care, and how people feel about others' access to care in time of need, the assumption of no externalities does not hold. Persons who are unable or who otherwise decline to purchase health insurance impose costs on other members of society. They may postpone care until illness has reached a stage that is more costly to treat, and they may rely on public sources of care due to lack of insurance or other means to pay for care (Pauly et. al. 1992). Thus, allocative efficiency may be enhanced by publicly mandating or providing coverage for services with proven effectiveness. However, publicly administered pricing under a single-payer, governmentally managed system may or may not lead to greater overall efficiency.

Each proposal attempts to achieve universal health care coverage, but the NHP is the only one that statutorily mandates coverage for the population. The PCP and CCHP use employer mandates and tax incentives for workers, and large subsidies for low-income persons and those not in the labor force to encourage enrollment in qualified health plans.

Equity. According to the criterion of equality of opportunity of access, those proposals that cover *everyone* in a *similar* fashion are deemed the fairest because they minimize the disparities in the type and extent of coverage, and the associated access differentials, that have been widely documented to exist—particularly between the publicly and privately insured. In addition, the promulgation of more-universal methods of coverage would reduce the increasing tendency of the private health insurance market to exclude or limit coverage for high-risk individuals—who are likely to need it the most.

The NHP proposal rates the highest in terms of the similar-treatment norm as this proposal treats everyone equally in terms of health insurance coverage. The CCHP proposal fares least well in terms of this criterion. The NHP proposal provides universal and comparable coverage, enrolling everyone in a single national insurance program. The CCHP and PCP proposals continue to promote dual public and private systems of care and coverage. Each of these proposals does, however, provide a basic minimum norm of coverage.

3. What is the basis for determining coverage?

Description

Consumer sovereignty, as revealed in market decisions, is the market-maximizing strategy used to determine health benefit coverage under the CCHP. The amount of employer subsidies would be based on the cost of a minimal benefits package similar to that included in the HMO Act: acute care, drug and alcohol abuse treatment, home care, certain preventive health services, and limited mental health services. Individuals would be allowed to choose the minimum benefit plan or another more costly plan to meet their needs. The competing view relies on need criteria determined by professionals and the community to define a benefit package for all. This approach is reflected in the NHP. All "medically necessary" services, as defined by experts, would be covered including: acute care, rehabilitation, prescription drugs, long-term care, home care, mental health services, dental care, occupational health services, medical supplies, and preventive and public health measures. Under the PCP, employer-offered plans and the national plan must meet minimum benefit requirements defined as "similar to but less generous than" the coverage most employers now offer. More costly plans may also be offered.

Evaluation

Effectiveness. Recognizing research that shows medical-care makes only a modest contribution to the health of the population, the population perspective on effectiveness indicates that society limit the use of resources for medical care and increase the level of investment in other health-producing services. Policy based on this perspective might include expanded support for: health protection (e.g., toxic agent control, occupational safety and health, fluoridation of community water supplies, infectious agent control); health promotion (e.g., smoking cessation, reducing misuse of alcohol and drugs, improved nutrition, exercise and fitness); investments in research and education on environmental and lifestyle factors related to health; and investments in preventive health services (e.g., family planning, prenatal and infant care, immunizations, sexually transmissible disease services). While the UHI proposals address some of the specific findings from research regarding medical care effectiveness, they offer little in terms of limiting overall system capacity and investing in preventive, protective, and promotive activities.

The clinical effectiveness perspective dictates that health insurance cover those services that have been shown to be effective in reducing morbidity and mortality of the population. Although additional research is needed, appropriateness-of-care guidelines could be developed for the 200 or so procedures that constitute most of medical practice (Brook 1991). Ideally, the United States should have an insurance plan that covers "necessary" care for all. The PCP and CCHP fall short of this criterion by defining basic coverage in terms of existing plans, the former on the average commercial plan and the latter on HMO plans. The NHP would be most likely to move the system toward funding the provision of appropriate care, since coverage provisions are to be based on evidence of appropriateness, and formal mechanisms (medical review boards) are proposed to ensure that practice patterns coincide with agreed-upon standards of appropriateness. Further, the methods of cost control, fee schedules, and global budgeting proposed by the NHP have been shown to work in other countries. Thus, this proposal may succeed better in constraining cost, saving funds for investment in structural and behavioral programs that may have more effect on health.

Efficiency. The choice of coverage depends on value orientation. People generally differ as to preference for risk and insurance coverage. As noted earlier, such preferences can lead to decisions that impose costs on others. Consequently, for services meeting basic needs, the role of consumer preferences must be minimized. However, for services beyond a basic minimum, consumer preferences should be considered in order to achieve allocative efficiency. Market-minimized approaches to health care are based on the concept of need as defined by health professionals. The object is to satisfy the most need, given the available resources. The NHP is a needs-based approach to universal coverage, whereas the PCP and CCHP balance need and demand in determining the type and extent of insurance coverage. The CCHP has the most clearly defined role for consumers in determining their needs and the shape of the future health care system.

Equity. Health services research has played and can continue to play a role in evaluating the types of services and care that are essential to improved outcomes. A decent, basic minimum of core benefits recognizes the continuum of preventive, acute, and long-term care that best meets medical care needs. The benefits provided under different plans vary a great deal with respect to the scope and depth of coverage. All three proposals acknowledge the importance of, and encourage, outcomes- and effectiveness-oriented research. Other than the explicit extension of coverage for preventive-oriented services in each of the plans, none seems to clearly discriminate what services might be the most efficacious.

The CCHP proposes the most restrictive set of benefits and the PCP the most comprehensive. The NHP offers the most promise of a decent, basic minimum based on need by covering what are deemed medically necessary services, which also presumably includes preventive and long-term care, though the exact nature of these benefits is not clearly defined.

4. What is the basis for determining payment methods and prices?

Description

The methods for determining payment methods range from government-determined, uniform payment rates and global budgets to a variety of methods that result from competition among insurers. The NHP proposes that expenditure limits be established by the government in cooperation with providers at the national and state levels. Physicians would be paid on a fee-for-service basis with an annually negotiated fee schedule. Providers such as hospitals, nursing homes, clinics, group practices, and home care agencies would receive a global budget, annually negotiated with each state's national-health-plan payment board. Under the PCP, Medicare policies for payment to hospitals and physicians would be expanded to apply to a broader segment of the population. Under the CCHP, providers would be paid in different ways based on the discretion of competing health plans. The authors of the CCHP predict that competitive plans will most likely adopt performance-based methods somewhere between fee-for-service and capitation.

Evaluation

Effectiveness. If medical guidelines are to be used to make care more effective, then previous research suggests that changing provider behavior will require both education and financial incentives. Financial incentives could include not reimbursing for inappropriate or equivocal services or rewarding the provision of appropriate care. Unfortunately, none of the proposals explicitly addresses the issue of providing payment incentives to encourage the provision of appropriate care. The CCHP does specifically call for outcomes assessment according to the prevailing model and proposes a managed care approach with the possibility of such incentives. The PCP calls for outcomes assessment and the development of practice guidelines, but neglects financial incentives. The NHP would focus on macromanagement of capacity and budget at the system level first and, once this is successfully implemented, turn attention to issues related to clinical outcomes.

Efficiency. Both market-oriented and non-market-oriented systems may pay providers in several different ways including fee-for-service, budgets, capitation, and salary. The payments represent mechanisms, although at different levels of service aggregation. The issue is how the prices are determined and how often they are adjusted in response to changes in the scarcity of resources and the preferences of consumers. Prices may be set unilaterally by government fiat, by bilateral negotiation between payers and providers, or by the interplay of supply and demand forces in local markets. Price flexibility is the key element in market-oriented systems. By providing a superior trade-off between price and quality, providers can attract consumers and thereby increase profits at the expense of their competitors. By making choices based on the available prices and qualities, consumers can signal what maximizes their well-being and what they are able and willing to pay.

A major concern with reliance on market-determined prices is whether enough consumers or their proxies—employers or government payers—can learn enough about the qualitative and effectiveness aspects of health care to make good choices. In addition, if services are insured, consumers are induced to purchase more than the optimal level of services, i.e., they consume too much care with low marginal benefits because the price to consumers would be at or near zero.

Under a government-determined price system, prices are generally inflexible for long periods of time and may bear little relationship to the changing preferences and needs of consumers. Providers have no incentive to lower prices to attract more patients, although they may offer a higher-quality service for the same, centrally determined price.

Experience suggests that there is no optimal system for pricing health services. While most Western, developed countries, excluding the United States, have provided a degree of price control, they continue to search for better ways to increase efficiency and satisfy the ever-increasing demands of providers and patients. Several countries, including the United Kingdom, New Zealand, and the Netherlands, are inserting market mechanisms into their universal health care systems. It is too early to tell how the results will compare to the command-and-control form of regulation (i.e., global budgets, negotiated fees, and capital controls).

We can only conclude for the proposals being considered for the United States, that efficiency is an uncertain outcome for each of the three. Unfortunately, it comes down to which approach one "believes" is the most appropriate in the U.S. context. The NHP treats health care like a public utility and establishes administered prices and budgets. The CCHP favors managed care systems such as HMOs and allows the market to determine prices within strict insurance guidelines on rate setting and a set of minimum benefits. The PCP encourages market competition for private plans, and public cost control as developed by Medicare for the expanded public plan. Managed care is a key element under both the public and private sectors.

Equity. The similar-treatment criterion with respect to how providers are reimbursed relates to (1) using the same reimbursement rate regardless of who pays for care (private versus public insurer, for example); and (2) limiting or capping reimbursement across all providers.

One of the major dilemmas that has emerged with the current multitiered system of financing is the widely varying rates of reimbursement to providers by different payers. As mentioned in previous chapters, the rates of Medicaid reimbursement in some states are much lower than those of private insurers, which has resulted in a dramatic reduction in the number of providers who are willing to see Medicaid-eligible clients.

Medical care systems in other countries, such as Canada, use more macro- rather than micro-oriented approaches to limit reimbursement, through negotiating global budgets and fee schedules with providers and limiting the funds available for capital expenditures for facilities and equipment. The assumption underlying these and other methods of capping provider reimbursement, however, is that providers (primarily physicians), not patients, are the main generators of demand for costly medical care services (hospitalizations, high-technology procedures, tests, pharmaceuticals, and so on). Cost-containment incentives at the micro level may also be needed for providers. However, if these incentives are to be implemented fairly, in terms of the similar-treatment norm, they must be applied across all the payers (or players) that reimburse providers for care. Otherwise, incentives remain, as they do now, for providers to serve those who can pay their full asking price and to refuse to provide care for the rest—many of whom are the sickest *and* most vulnerable. (See also discussion of cost containment by all-payer systems relative to the efficiency discussion for criterion 8.)

The NHP proposal best implements these similar treatment norms for provider reimbursement. In contrast, the CCHP encourages market-determined variability across plans in the rates and ceilings for provider reimbursement. The PCP maintains the variation of the current, mixed system of provider reimbursement—requiring Medicare rules of provider reimbursement for those enrolled through the public plan but imposing no restrictions on those who are privately insured.

5. What is the extent of consumer copayments?

Description

Under the market-minimized approach of the NHP, there would be no copayments or deductibles. Consumer out-of-pocket costs play a strong role in the market-maximized approach. The consumer pays higher premium costs to enroll in more costly plans and deductibles and coinsurance for services. The PCP includes deductibles ($250 per individual and $500 per family) and coinsurance (20 percent for basic services and 50 percent for outpatient mental health services), subject to ability to pay. People below the poverty level pay no premiums, deductibles, or coinsurance. There would be limited subsidies for people with incomes up to twice the poverty standard. The CCHP proposes deductibles up to $250 per person and a coinsurance rate of 20 percent for middle- and upper-income groups. Individuals who select high-cost plans would pay higher premiums. Premium subsidies by employers would be fixed at 80 percent of the cost of a basic minimum plan. The premium copayment would be subsidized on a graduated basis for low-income persons.

Evaluation

Effectiveness. Copayments differentially reduce the use and benefits of health services for those with different incomes. In the RAND Health Insurance Experiment, it was found that "free" care did not result in improved health status for the average person compared to people with higher copayments and less utilization. This finding suggests that cost sharing may ration inappropriate care resulting from overuse by the middle class and upper class. However, for persons who were low-income and initially sick, "free" care resulted in improvement in blood pressure control and vision acuity compared to the copayment group (Manning et al. 1987). These findings suggest a targeted approach to copayments under UHI (see discussion relative to criterion 1 above).

The NHP ranks below the other two proposals in addressing this issue since it eliminates copayments for the entire population. The PCP and CCHP adopt a more-targeted approach by relating copayments to income.

Efficiency. Copayments are designed to sensitize patients to the cost of medical services and to reduce the transactions costs associated with small claims. Both of these outcomes should help restrain the expected losses and thereby the premiums associated with insurance policies. Copayments affect the demand side of the health care market and thus are expected to influence allocative efficiency. Insurance tends to reduce the price of service below its social cost and hence induces consumers to use services that have a marginal social cost greater than the marginal benefit, resulting in a welfare loss to society. Copayments restore price while still protecting consumers from losses beyond the copayment limit. The value of copayment must be weighed against the possible losses associated with reduction in protection against risk, and the negative health consequences associated with delay or reduction in health service use.

The RAND Health Insurance Experiment demonstrated that copayments have a substantial effect on health care utilization and expenditure. The welfare losses associated with copayment were estimated by examining the extent to which zero prices (no copayment) induced patients to consume services past the point at which the marginal benefit of a service equals the marginal cost. As reported in Chapter 4, findings documented a substantial welfare loss from first dollar coverage. Thus, the evidence suggests that the absence of copayments can lead the average consumer to substantial use of unnecessary care. However, it may still be prudent to minimize copayments for low-income households, especially given other barriers they may face in obtaining health services.

Both the CCHP and PCP allow the use of copayments in structuring insurance policies, while setting an annual copayment cap. The proposals also subsidize low-income persons to protect them from the negative consequences of copayments. The NHP follows the Canadian model and does not use copayment. Therefore, the NHP is less preferred than the other two plans on this criterion.

Equity. The burden of out-of-pocket costs for medical care has traditionally fallen most heavily on the low-income population, for whom even a relatively small dollar outlay may represent a substantial proportion of financial resources. Evidence from the RAND Health Insurance Experiment suggests that increased cost sharing may ration effective as well as less-effective care and may also differentially affect the access of those who either need it most or can least afford it.

The NHP proposes a minimal out-of-pocket burden on consumers, while the CCHP mandates that consumers pay 20 percent of the base-plan premium to motivate consumers to make cost-conscious choices among plans. The CCHP does impose a ceiling on out-of-pocket payments. The PCP also imposes ceilings on what consumers are expected to pay out-of-pocket.

6. How would it be financed?

Description

All financing would be through a combination of corporate and personal taxes in the market-minimized NHP. The other two proposals would be financed primarily through employer-employee premiums and out-of-pocket payments. Under the PCP, employers pay 80 percent of the premium for covered employees or an equivalent payroll tax to support the federal plan. Employed individuals pay a maximum of 20 percent of the premium for the public plan or may elect private coverage. Those not covered through employment would pay the full cost of the federal plan, subject to ability to pay. Under the CCHP, employers and public sponsors would pay 80 percent of the premium of a basic minimum health plan. The person or family covered would pay the difference between the employer or sponsor contribution and the cost of the plan they choose. Employers pay 8 percent payroll tax up to $22,500 for employees in public-sponsor plans; employees opting for the public plan must pay the difference between their sponsor's contribution and the cost of the plan they choose. Self-employed or unemployed individuals with income above the poverty level pay 8 percent personal income tax to support public-sponsor plans.

Evaluation

Effectiveness. The population perspective on effectiveness would argue for that mode of financing that is most likely to maximize the health of the population as a whole, while the clinical perspective would argue for the system that assures the provision of the most-effective care. The conceptual and empirical foundations for determing which of the specific proposals is most likely to assure these outcomes have been discussed previously. Overall, the effectiveness perspective cannot strongly endorse any of the specific proposals because of the uncertainty of the likely beneficial effects of each one's mode of financing.

Efficiency. Health services may be financed by taxes, insurance premiums, and copayments, or by some combination of those sources. Typically, taxes are progressive with respect to income and are unrelated to a person's health status or health care utilization. Insurance premiums can be either community- or experience-rated. Community-rated premiums are the same for the same benefits for everyone in a community, whereas experience-rated premiums depend on the health care utilization experience of groups or individuals. If insurance and its associated premiums are compulsory, there is little effective difference between taxes and premiums except that taxes are more directly related to ability to pay. The real issue is between community- and experience-rated systems. A tax system tends to be community-rated in that payments are not related to health care utilization experience.

From a consumer-sovereignty framework, Feldstein (1988) argues that community rating is allocatively inefficient. In such a system, high-risk persons or groups are subsidized by low-risk persons or groups. Community premiums or taxes will reflect the average expected claims plus administrative cost. This amount will likely be larger than what many low-risk groups or individuals are willing to pay for health insurance. Many of these people will choose not to purchase insurance. They are then worse off than if they could purchase an insurance program based on the cost of insurance (actuarial value plus an administrative fee).

Under community rating the low-risk groups are essentially paying a tax to cover the cost of insuring the high-risk groups. As in other markets, this distorts the decisions consumers make, and they purchase less than would be efficient. If forced to participate, low-risk persons will consume a service whose value is less than its cost to them. Because of consumer preferences to pay no more than the cost of production, community-rated systems are less desired when the focus is on trying to create competitive health insurance markets. This becomes even more problematic when consumers have different preferences with respect to benefits and levels of copayment. It is very difficult to design a community rate that can accommodate these preferences.

Glaser (1991) found that most statutory health insurance plans, such as those in western Europe and Canada, rely on payroll taxes rather than premiums for financing. Initially, taxes were allowed to rise to cover increases in health care costs, but as cost and deficit problems occurred in the 1970s, governments constrained tax increases in order to curb the funds going into health care. This approach to cost containment has been more effective than the U.S. attempt to micromanage health care costs in a system with hundreds of payers and no effective global revenue control.

From the consumer-sovereignty perspective, payroll tax financing may lead to inefficient allocation of resources to health insurance and medical care services compared to a competitive market that prices insurance according to actual cost. In the absence of a workable, competitive insurance and health care market, payroll taxes provide societal control over the resources going into health care, which otherwise may be excessive, given the dominance of providers. Thus, a payroll-tax statutory system may offer a second-best solution.

The NHP offers such an approach to health care financing and therefore has the potential to constrain total cost. However, within this proposal physicians are given great latitude to allocate resources within the macro constraints. Allocative efficiency will depend on how well physicians act as agents for patients to maximize their well-being. Given that the NHP proposes first dollar coverage and fee-for-service payment of physicians, achievement of efficiency under that proposal is problematic.

The CCHP has a combination of private insurance premiums and taxes to finance universal health care. It requires the availability of a standardized minimum benefit package, open enrollment, and community rating by actuarial category in order to provide incentives for health plans to enroll high-risk groups. To address equity concerns, beneficiaries are also subsidized according to their actuarial category. The unproven promise of the CCHP is that it creates a workable competitive health care market that has the potential to allow consumer choice to determine the amount of resources spent on health care and the type of services provided. It also provides incentives for providers to minimize the cost of production. Efficiency therefore depends on how well the system actually works once in place, and this is very difficult to gauge beforehand.

While the PCP reforms the underwriting and risk-rating practices of the private health insurance market, and converts Medicaid to a nonwelfare public program to include all the poor, it does not offer fundamental reform of the health care market nor does it provide global controls on health care spending. Financing would continue to be a combination of job-based private-insurance premiums and taxes to support the public program. While the plan encourages consumer choice among managed care plans, fundamental tax incentives are not altered to make consumers cost-conscious. Tax credits would subsidize insurance purchases by small businesses. The Pepper Commission suggests a combination of specific and general tax sources to finance the program but does not make a specific recommendation.

Equity. The major criterion in evaluating the fairness of financing with respect to the similar treatment norm is the use of community-based risk sharing and progressive patient contributions. Community rating refers to the fact that the basis for computing actuarial risks and the attendant effect on premiums is based on broad, rather than narrow, population groupings. Experience rating, in contrast, bases rates on a narrowly defined group of eligibles, providing incentives to limit eligibility and enrollment to those who are likely to require the least-expensive care, to keep the price of premiums down. The result is that those most in need (those with serious health problems or who are at risk of developing them, such as persons who test positive for the human immunodeficiency virus) are likely to be excluded or charged very high rates for coverage.

The NHP rates highest in terms of the universality norm, and both the PCP and NHP demonstrate a commitment to broadening the basis for computing and sharing risks. The CCHP fares least well in terms of both the universality and community-rating criteria.

The NHP proposal provides universal and comparable coverage, since everyone would be enrolled in one national insurance program. The CCHP and PCP continue to promote dual public and private systems of care and coverage. The PCP also proposes that the private health insurance industry be reformed to require premiums based on community rating. The CCHP proposes community rating, but allows different rates for high-risk consumers.

The NHP proposes the most progressive method of financing care through payroll, income, or other progressive taxes, with a minimal out-of-pocket burden on consumers, while the CCHP mandates that consumers pay 20 percent of the base plan premium as a basis for motivating cost-conscious consumer choices among plans. The proposal does impose ceilings on out-of-pocket payments. The PCP also requires consumers to pay a portion of premiums and imposes ceilings on what consumers are expected to pay out-of-pocket.

7. How would it be administered?

Description

Administration options for the three proposals range from a single government administrator to multiple private insurers. In the middle are either multiple (state-level) government administrators, a limited number of private insurers regulated by the federal government, or both. Under the NHP, one government agency within each state would establish caps, set payment rates, and process claims, subject to national standards. A local planning process would be used to approve capital expenditures.

Major employers either purchase private coverage for employees or pay a tax to support a newly established federal plan under the PCP. The federal plan would be administered in conjunction with, or as a part of, Medicare and would replace Medicaid. There would be national standards for eligibility, benefits, and payment. Under the CCHP, public sponsors and employers serve as insurance brokers, selecting a variety of health plans to be offered, managing the enrollment process, collecting premiums, and paying providers. Medicare and Medicaid would remain the same.

Evaluation

Effectiveness. None of the plans offers an administrative framework for improving the population's health. The NHP proposes to set spending caps on services and to control capital expenditures. What is not clear is the derivation of those limits, that is, there is no specification for developing a national health policy. The CCHP relies on unproven market incentives as well as practice guidelines for coverage and control. The PCP falls between these two with its public and employer-based plans for insuring the coverage of the population. It appears to lack any overall financial controls or planning efforts.

Efficiency. Administration represents over 20 percent of U.S. health care expenditures; how programs are administered has important implications for production efficiency. Research shows that there are economies of scale in the provision of insurance services, suggesting that larger firms are more efficient than smaller firms, but it does not imply that costs fall continually as size expands. The Canadian single-payer system, however, administered by province, is about one-half as expensive to administer as the U.S. model of multiple programs (General Accounting Office 1991). This implies that substantial savings can be achieved by a simplified single-payer program compared to the complexity of hundreds of payers attempting to market, monitor, and service health insurance and health care delivery programs in the United States.

There is no inherent advantage to one type of system in terms of the efficiency by which health services are provided. Efficiency depends on the costs of administration relative to outputs achieved. Much U.S. health care administration is aimed at improving the quality of care, assuring that appropriate care is delivered, and that consumers have insurance products that address their individual risk and preferences for insurance and medical services. We currently know very little about how well administrative investments achieve these goals (Thorpe 1992).

The approach to improving outcome (quality) and minimizing the inefficiency of production methods is to encourage cost-based and quality-based competition under the CCHP model, and to control prices and the level, mix, and location of resources in the single-payer NHP model. The CCHP model has not been proven. The NHP model may contain cost by funneling payment through a few channels, but does not necessarily result in more-efficient modes of service delivery or better quality of care. However, given current evidence, savings from administrative efficiency provides an important rationale for the single-payer model.

Equity. The freedom-of-choice norm, as applied to evaluating the equity consequences of UHI proposals, may be judged by what a proposal requires with respect to limiting consumers' choice of care. Those proposals that minimize the constraints on consumers' choices would be the fairest, according to this criterion.

What each of the three proposals fails to acknowledge fully is that consumers' choices over the types of medical care they ultimately receive are, in general, limited—in either the market-minimized or the market-maximized approach. In either case, the physician acts as the patients' agent in deciding what care is likely to be best for them. The main discretion consumers have over the care they ultimately receive is a function of the choices they have of the providers they can see in the first place. The more doors that are closed to consumers because of the unavailability of providers in an area or the unwillingness of providers to see patients with certain types of coverage, the closed-panel nature of medical practice, or the lack of an informed knowledge basis for choosing among providers, the fewer the effective choices that are available to consumers. None of the three proposals for universal health insurance is likely to enhance greatly the choices consumers have in the U.S. medical care marketplace.

The CCHP encourages the formation and promulgation of managed care plans (e.g., HMOs, PPOs), which are assumed to be the most cost-effective competitors for employers' and the public's business in a given market area. Consumers' choices would be constrained by the plans that emerge in the area, in response to incentives provided by public and private sponsors in each state for the development of such plans. Further, the CCHP does not directly provide for Medicare- and Medicaid-eligible individuals, so it is not clear what options would ultimately be available to those individuals that providers may be least inclined to serve. One may presume the options would be the same as now, which in many cases includes access to HMOs.

The PCP encourages, but does not mandate, the promulgation of managed care alternatives. It also encourages the delivery of services to underserved areas. The focus of the NHP is principally on altering the method of *paying for, not providing,* care. The NHP neither suggests nor requires changes in the existing delivery system, which, as noted earlier, continues to limit the effective alternatives available to many of the vulnerable. An improvement for equity is that physicians would be paid the same rates by rich and poor alike. That will not eliminate the geographical distribution problem, but it should help.

8. How would costs be controlled?

Description

Under the market-minimizing approach of the NHP, cost control would be achieved through negotiated fees and global budgets for providers and a planning process for capital expenditures. Under the PCP, the publicly administered plan would rely on generous coverage of preventive services and would utilize Medicare payment methods (e.g., DRGs for hospital inpatient care) to control cost. Private plans would be encouraged to use managed care and cost sharing to enhance consumer sensitivity to the cost of medical services. The CCHP relies on consumer sovereignty and market dynamics (the interaction of supply and demand) to create incentives for cost control. Consumers would be made cost-conscious by the requirement that they pay 20 percent of the average cost of the basic plan plus any additional cost associated with the plan they choose. While employee benefits might cover these costs, the benefits would be subject to income tax. Regulated health plans would be required to compete on the basis of price and quality and not by preferred risk selection. The government would be responsible for disseminating information about providers' prices and quality of services, and new insurance structures would be developed to encourage competition.

Evaluation

Effectiveness. To the degree that an attempt will be made to modify the practice of medicine under any UHI proposal, then the research findings about practice guidelines become relevant. In fact, repeated studies have shown that dissemination of practice guidelines alone does little to alter the behavior of providers (Hill, Levine, and Whelton 1988; Kosecoff, Kanouse, and Rogers 1987; Lomas et al. 1989; and Wennberg 1984). However, when combined with the financial incentives that are suggested by the UHI proposals, practice guidelines can alter behavior. The analysis of these provisions is covered in criterion 7, above. The NHP plan is favored because its macromanagement strategy for cost control is more likely to result in care being based on clinical principles and resources being available for investment in programs that have the potential to improve community health (Brook 1991). Both clinical and economic principles must be applied in order to achieve the most health improvement for a given amount of resources (Culyer 1992).

Efficiency. There is universal concern in developed countries that the health care system is consuming resources that would yield more value if invested in other social or private endeavors. This concern is expressed in the desire to contain health care costs. Single-payer systems or those that funnel payment through relatively few channels and rely on community planning to control expensive technology are the only ones that demonstrate an ability to limit cost increases to the growth in income in the country. The U.S. model of multiple payers is a notable failure in limiting cost increases. However, cost control cannot be equated with efficiency. Limiting expenditure does not necessarily result in lowering the cost of production or attaining the right, most-valued mix of goods and services. Arbitrary cost control may lead to less well-being by restricting useful services and by retarding innovation in the delivery of health care. Similarly, without a well-functioning market, lack of controls may lead to expansion of services with low marginal value relative to cost and to lack of effort to utilize efficient production methods. The question is which system provides the second-best solution to health care resource allocation. Clearly, from the narrow perspective of cost control, the planning-and-budget-control policy has the most empirical support to date. As mentioned above, some countries that have traditionally relied on planning and budgeting are now introducing competitive processes. The Netherlands, the United Kingdom, and New Zealand have a hybrid of supply-side competition within the context of an overall budget. It is too early to judge the performance of this approach.

The NHP will utilize public-utility-style regulation of prices and capital to control cost, whereas the CCHP will use market competition between health plans. The PCP will use a combination of consumer cost sharing, competition among plans, and government cost controls. Empirical evidence is lacking on which approach may best achieve the goals of allocative and production efficiency in the U.S. political and cultural context.

Equity. Evidence from other countries that impose limits on the rates of reimbursement across providers, as well as from states that have all-payer systems of reimbursement, demonstrates their greater success in controlling health care costs. This is also a fairer basis for cost containment since it minimizes provider *disincentives* to treat certain (e.g., Medicaid, Medicare) patients differently because of different levels of reimbursement. Further, since providers are often the major "consumers" of expensive, technology-intensive care (acting as the patient's agent), incentives to reduce their "excess" consumption are also warranted.

The NHP offers the most promise—theoretically—of containing the costs of care through providing a single-payer system with universally applied standards for determining global budgets and fee schedules. The Canadian health care system (on which the NHP was modeled) is currently considering replacing its system of reimbursing the majority of physicians on a fee-for-service basis with salary or capitation methods. Through enrolling all providers and consumers in an area in competing health plans, the CCHP would theoretically reduce expenditures for care by encouraging consumers to become more-prudent purchasers and by providing incentives for physicians to practice more cost-effective medicine. The health services research evidence from other countries, as well as from all-payer states in the United States, argues for the probable success of the NHP model, while the findings regarding the lower utilization of expensive and intensive (in particular, hospital) services in HMOs, tends to support the CCHP, though the evidence is weaker on the systemwide or marketwide cost savings of competition. The PCP does little to alter the current system of reimbursing health care providers and containing costs.

Summary

The analyses point out both the convergence and conflict among the goals of effectiveness, efficiency, and equity that are suggested by the three proposals (see Figure 9.1). With respect to coverage provisions—who is covered, how they are covered, and the basis for determining coverage—the market-minimizing provisions of the NHP are generally favored. The NHP is rated highest on all three provisions in terms of its prospects for achieving equity. The NHP best meets efficiency criteria for who is covered because of its use of mandates for necessary services, which would minimize external costs of noncoverage. However, the PCP and CCHP are preferred for allowing a role for consumer choice in determining coverage for services beyond those required to meet basic needs. The population perspective on effectiveness is critical of all three proposals because they fail to address adequately the health trade-offs between medical and nonmedical health-producing services. This perspective is also critical of the NHP because it does not provide greater incentives for low-income groups to obtain needed services.

The proposed market-minimizing strategies of the NHP for provider payment and price determination are also favored from the equity perspective. However, the proposal's lack of financial incentives for appropriate care is a problem in terms of ensuring effectiveness and efficiency. Furthermore, the potential inflexibility of government-determined prices raises efficiency concerns as the preferences and needs of consumers change over time.

Equity criteria favor the NHP over the other two proposals with respect to its copayment provisions. The lack of copayments for middle- and upper-income groups would likely result in an allocation of resources that is both ineffective and inefficient, however. Efficiency research on the demand effects of full coverage point to the potential for excessive use under such a proposal, resulting in utilization of services with little or no marginal benefit (ineffective services).

With respect to financing strategies, the efficiency perspective favors the CCHP approach of combining private insurance premiums, copayments, and taxes to create the potential for a competitive marketplace. This strategy falls short with respect to equity, however, which favors the NHP because of its more-progressive financing methods of taxation and minimal out-of-pocket payments.

All three perspectives are equivocal with respect to the administrative provisions of the proposals. None of the plans specifically addresses the population health goals of the effectiveness perspective in its administrative provisions. Existing evidence points to advantages and disadvantages of government- and privately administered plans in terms of achieving efficiency. The comparisons between the Canadian and U.S. systems in terms of administrative cost tell only half the story since they do not compare the costs to outputs achieved. The equity objective of freedom of choice is not adequately addressed by any of the proposals. Choices over the types of medical care that consumers ultimately are likely to receive are, in general, limited in both the market-minimized and market-maximized strategies.

The cost-control provisions of the NHP are favored by both the effectiveness and equity perspectives. Health services research from other countries, as well as from all-payer states in the United States, provide support for the cost-containing effect of the NHP provisions. The effectiveness evaluation is more conceptual, based on the argument that global budgeting and capital controls are more likely to cap the system and allow attention to be focused on clinical outcomes. The efficiency perspective is equivocal on this provision. While noting the cost-containment potential of the NHP, empirical evidence is lacking on whether a market-minimizing or market-maximizing approach may best achieve the goals of allocative and production efficiency.

This analysis demonstrates that none of the proposed strategies consistently optimizes any of these objectives, though the single-payer NHP proposal does tend to fare best on most of the equity indicators. The results also reveal the trade-offs among the objectives represented in the proposals. They also reflect the ambiguities, lack of specificity, and gaps in knowledge of the consequences, of selected provisions that must be addressed to make effective judgments of their probable impact.

The evidence and arguments presented also pose challenges to some of the traditional assumptions governing the performance of the U.S. medical care system with respect to the effectiveness, efficiency, and equity. Rationing care on the basis of price (consumer copayments) does not, on average, lead to reductions in the provision of *needed* care. Government-regulated prices and expenditure caps that reduce cost do not necessarily result in *more-efficient* service provision. The promulgation of an array of competing health insurance plans does not inevitably give rise to *more* consumer choice in the medical care marketplace.

For many years the debate over the need for and type of universal health insurance program has revolved around the consequences of competing financing strategies. Health services research can assist in framing current and future policy debates on this issue by clarifying the goals, trade-offs, and assumptions of alternative proposals based on the valued system-performance criteria of effectiveness, efficiency, and equity.

Conclusion

The discussion in this and previous chapters examines the conceptual and normative blueprints of the major health care system goals of effectiveness, efficiency, and equity. It analyzes the balance and trade-offs resulting in designing policies and programs to realize these objectives. It reviews the methods to measure the extent to which each of these goals has actually been achieved. And it encourages dialogue among health services researchers, policy analysts, policymakers, and administrators— who study, recommend, formulate, and implement health policy. Designing a health care system that optimizes the policy ideals of effectiveness, efficiency, and equity requires critical inquiry into the meaning of these goals and how best to achieve them. This book seeks to invite such inquiry.

References

Brook, R. 1991. "Health, Health Insurance, and the Uninsured." *Journal of the American Medical Association* 265: 2998–3002.

Brown, E. 1988. "Principles for a National Health Program: A Framework for Analysis and Development." *Milbank Quarterly* 66: 573–617.

Culyer, A. 1992. "The Morality of Efficiency in Health Care—Some Uncomfortable Implications." *Health Economics* 1: 7–18.

Enthoven, A., and R. Kronick. 1989a. "A Consumer-Choice Health Plan for the 1990s: Universal Health Insurance in a System Designed to Promote Quality and Economy." *New England Journal of Medicine* 320: 29–37.

———. 1989b. "A Consumer-Choice Health Plan for the 1990s: Universal Health Insurance in a System Designed to Promote Quality and Economy." *New England Journal of Medicine* 320: 94–101.

———. 1991. "Universal Health Insurance through Incentives Reform." *Journal of the American Medical Association* 265: 2532–36.

Feldstein, P. 1988. *Health Care Economics*, 3rd ed. NY: John Wiley & Sons.

General Accounting Office. 1991. *Canadian Health Insurance: Lessons for the United States*. GAO/HRD-91-90. Washington, DC: U.S. General Accounting Office.

Glaser, W. 1991. *Health Insurance in Practice*. San Francisco: Jossey-Bass.

Grumbach, K., T. Bodenheimer, D. Himmelstein, and S. Woolhandler. 1991. "Liberal Benefits, Conservative Spending: The Physicians for a National Health Program Proposal." *Journal of the American Medical Association.* 265: 2549–54.

Hill, M., D. Levine, and P. Whelton. 1988. "Awareness, Use and Impact of the 1984 Joint National Committee Consensus Report on High Blood Pressure." *American Journal of Public Health* 78: 1190–94.

Himmelstein, D., S. Woolhandler, and the Writing Committee of the Working Group on Program Design. 1989. "A National Health Program for the United States: A Physicians' Proposal." *New England Journal of Medicine* 320: 102–8.

Hollingsworth, J. 1981. "Inequality in Levels of Health in England and Wales." *Journal of Health and Social Behavior* 22: 268–83.

Kosecoff, J., D. Kanouse, and W. Rogers. 1987. "Effects of the National Institutes of Health Consensus Development Program on Physician Practice." *Journal of the American Medical Association* 258: 2708–13.

Lomas, J., G. Anderson, K. Domnick-Pierre, E. Vayda, M. Enkin, and W. Hannah. 1989. "Do Practice Guidelines Guide Practice? The Effect of a Consensus Statement on the Practice of Physicians." *New England Journal of Medicine* 321: 1306–11.

Manning, W., J. Newhouse, N. Duan, E. Keeler, A. Leibowitz, and S. Marquis. 1987. "Health Insurance and the Demand for Medical Care: Evidence from a Randomized Experiment." *American Economic Review* 77 (3): 251–77.

Pauly, M., P. Danzon, P. Feldstein, and J. Hoff. 1992. *Responsible National Health Insurance*. Washington, DC: American Enterprise Institute.

Pepper Commission: U.S. Bipartisan Commission on Comprehensive Health Care. 1990. *A Call for Action: Final Report*. Washington, DC: U.S. Government Printing Office.

Somers, A., and H. Somers. 1977. "A Proposed Framework for Health and Health Care Policies." *Inquiry* 14: 115–70.

Thorpe, K. 1992. "Inside the Black Box of Administrative Costs." *Health Affairs* 11: 41–55.

Wennberg, J. 1984. "Dealing with Medical Practice Variations: A Proposal for Action." *Health Affairs* 3: 6–32.

Index

Access: actual, 140–41, 142–43; alternative solutions, 150–51; analytic research, 133; descriptive research, 132–33; evaluative research, 133; financing, 144–45; health insurance problems, 149–50; and medical care financing, 143–45; mental health care, 142; patient satisfaction and, 132; and population outcomes, 51–52; potential, 140. *See also* Equity of access

Access indicators: cost effectiveness, 130–31; decent, basic minimum, 129; freedom of choice, 127–28; need, 130; similar treatment, 128–29

Accountability: release of hospital mortality statistics, 26

Acquired immune deficiency syndrome. *See* AIDS

Acute Physiology and Chronic Health Evaluation (APACHE): risk adjustment, 39

Administration: universal health insurance proposals, 200–203

AFDC. *See* Aid to Families with Dependent Children

African-Americans: life expectancy, 24; utilization and, 17, 147

Agency for Health Care Policy and Research (AHCPR), 10, 64; clinical guidelines, 62; medical practice guidelines, 27; National Medical Care Expenditure surveys access studies, 135; Patient Outcome Research Team (PORT), 60–61, 62–63, 131; outcomes assessment and management, 58–59

AHA. *See* American Hospital Association

AHCPR. *See* Agency for Health Care Policy and Research

AHSR. *See* Association for Health Services Research

AIDS, 12; mortality, 24

Aid to Families with Dependent Children (AFDC): access problems, 150

AIMS. *See* Arthritis Impact Measurement Scale

Allocative efficiency, 76, 99–104; evaluating, 91–92; problems, 73

AMA. *See* American Medical Association

Ambulatory services: utilization, 16–17

American College of Cardiology, 63

American College of Obstetricians and Gynecologists: practice guidelines, 63

About the Authors

Lu Ann Aday, Ph.D., is Professor of Behavioral Sciences and Management and Policy Sciences at the University of Texas School of Public Health. She received her doctorate in sociology from Purdue University, and was formerly Associate Director for Research at the Center for Health Administration Studies of the University of Chicago. Dr. Aday's principal research interests have focused on indicators and correlates of health services utilization and access. She has conducted major national and community surveys and evaluations of national demonstrations and published extensively in this area, including nine previous books dealing with conceptual or empirical aspects of research on equity of access to medical care.

Charles E. Begley, Ph.D., is Associate Professor of Management and Policy Sciences at the University of Texas School of Public Health and a member of the adjunct faculty in the Department of Economics at Rice University. He received his doctorate in economics from the University of Texas at Austin and has been on the faculty of Sangamon State University and Southern Illinois University School of Medicine in Springfield, Illinois. Dr. Begley's research and teaching interests include the economic evaluation of health care programs and health policy analysis, and he has conducted policy analyses of an array of state-level policy proposals and programs.

David R. Lairson, Ph.D., is Professor of Health Economics on the faculty of the University of Texas School of Public Health and a member of the adjunct faculty in the Department of Economics at Rice University. This book was completed while he was on leave as Adjunct Professor on the faculty of Queensland University of Technology, School of Public Health in Brisbane, Australia. He was a doctoral fellow at the Kaiser Center for Health Research in Portland, Oregon, and received his Ph.D. from the University of Kentucky in Lexington, Kentucky. Dr. Lairson's major research and teaching interests include the economic evaluation of health care programs and services and the organization and financing of health care systems.

Carl H. Slater, M.D., is Associate Professor of Health Services Organization on the faculty of the University of Texas School of Public Health. He is a graduate of the University of Colorado School of Medicine, and was a Fellow at the Center for the Study of Medical Education, University of Illinois, School of Medicine in Chicago. Dr. Slater's research interests are in assessing the quality and effectiveness of medical care, with a special emphasis on ambulatory care programs in the public sector. Dr. Slater has developed and taught courses in health services effectiveness, quality assessment, and outcomes assessment; published in the area of ambulatory care quality assessment; and edited a special issue of *Evaluation and the Health Professions* on outcomes assessment.